praise for
make your own rules diet

"Tara's laid-back, fun approach to yoga and cooking is a refreshing relief!
She makes healthy living both accessible and enjoyable. I am a huge fan of her work
and adore her latest book, *Make Your Own Rules Diet*. Check it out!"

—KRIS CARR,
New York Times best-selling author of *Crazy Sexy Kitchen*

"The key to true wellness, many of us are finding, is so very much about finding your own way.
With so many competing messages bombarding us, this can be nigh impossible to do and
many of us have simply lost our wellness mojo. Tara's approach, however, shows how real, lasting
wellness is about being gentle and kind, shifting with ease, and creating space (my mantra
for my own wellness is all about creating space—in my schedule and also at a cellular level).
Make Your Own Rules Diet is a genuine handbook for a real wellness shift."

—SARAH WILSON,
New York Times best-selling author of *I Quit Sugar*

"This is a fantastic book! Tara Stiles effortlessly teaches you how to use a yoga mat, a meditation
cushion, and your kitchen to transform your body into the one you have always desired.
The program is stress-free, fun, and easy! Enjoy your personal journey to wellness!"

—DR. RUDY TANZI,
New York Times best-selling author of *Super Brain*, professor of
neurology at Harvard Medical School, and director, Genetics and Aging
Research Unit MassGeneral Institute for Neurodegenerative Disease

"I live and work in a world that's fast paced and focuses on perfection. I'm surrounded by it every day.
Tara has taught me to embrace my imperfections, love all of me, and embrace all that makes me happy.
More important, she's taught me life is a journey, not a race; slow down and go at your own pace. It's okay."

—TIA MOWRY,
actress and CEO of Need Brands

"Vibrant health is not a destination, but the journey of our lifetime. So how about we drop the dogma,
judgments, and worry so we can make this journey as fun, pleasurable, and exciting as possible?
Tara teaches you how with her practical tips, loving encouragement, and contagious enthusiasm.
This isn't just a book; it's a liberating experience."

—JESSICA ORTNER,
New York Times best-selling author of *The Tapping Solution for Weight Loss and Body Confidence*

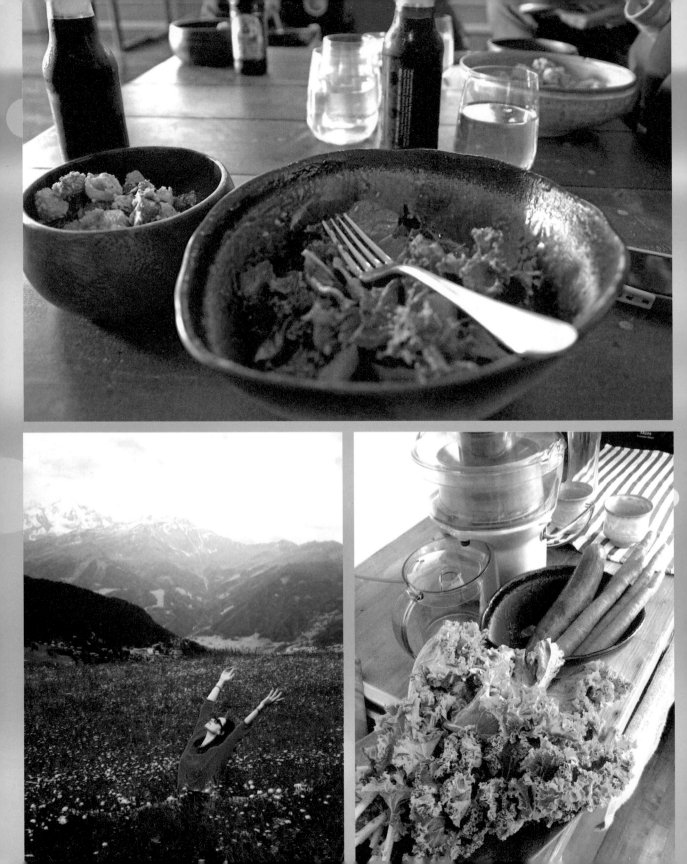

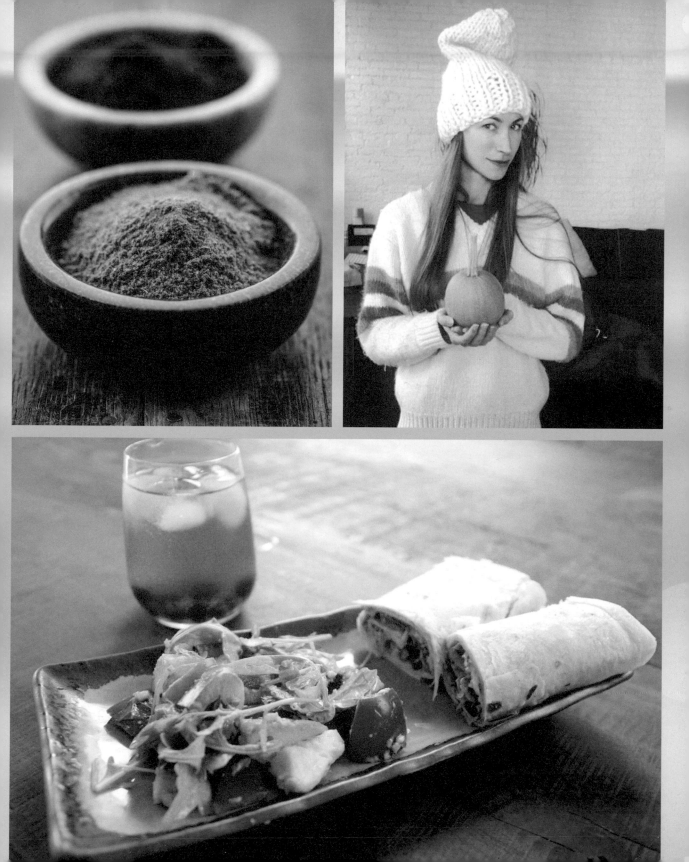

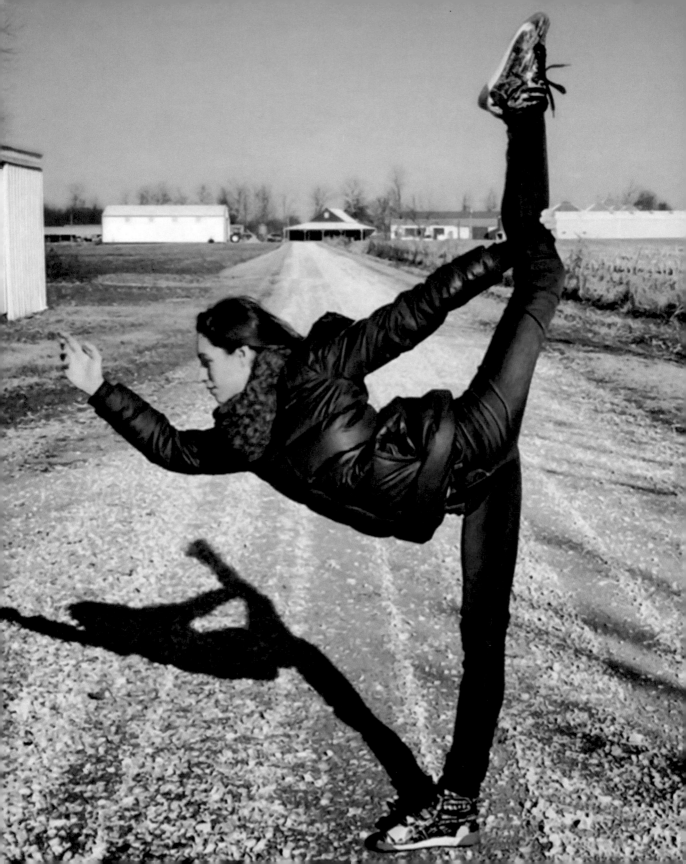

make
your
own
rules
diet

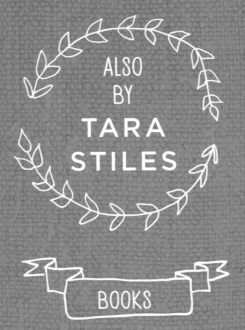

ALSO BY TARA STILES

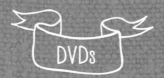

BOOKS

Slim Calm Sexy Yoga:
210 Proven Yoga Moves for Mind/Body Bliss

Yoga Cures: Simple Routines to Conquer
More Than 50 Ailments and Live Pain-Free

DVDs

Jane Fonda's Workout:
Daily Yoga with Tara Stiles

Tia Mowry's Calm & Core Yoga Series with Tara Stiles

This Is Yoga

Yoga Transformation Series (with Deepak Chopra)

TARA STILES

make your own rules diet

HAY HOUSE, INC.

Carlsbad, California   New York City
London   Sydney   Johannesburg
Vancouver   Hong Kong   New Delhi

Published and distributed in the United States by: Hay House, Inc.: www.hayhouse.com
Published and distributed in Australia by: Hay House Australia Pty. Ltd.: www.hayhouse.com.au
Published and distributed in the United Kingdom by: Hay House UK, Ltd.: www.hayhouse.co.uk
Published and distributed in the Republic of South Africa by: Hay House SA (Pty.), Ltd.: www.hayhouse.co.za
Distributed in Canada by: Raincoast Books: www.raincoast.com
Published in India by: Hay House Publishers India: www.hayhouse.co.in

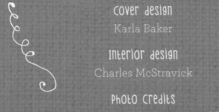

Cover design
Karla Baker

Interior design
Charles McStravick

Photo credits
Photo on title page by Ryan Kibler

Photos on pages 168, 180, 184, 188, 192, 202, 210, 216, 222, 226,
230, 234, 238, 242, 246, and 250 by Andrew Scrivani

All other photos courtesy of Tara Stiles

Library of Congress Cataloging-in-Publication Data

Stiles, Tara.
    Make your own rules diet / Tara Stiles.
       pages cm
    ISBN 978-1-4019-4435-3 (hardback)
    1. Self-control. 2. Yoga. 3. Diet. I. Title.
    BF632.S75 2014
    613--dc23

                                                    2014012500

Hardcover ISBN: 978-1-4019-4435-3

10 9 8 7 6 5 4 3 2
1st edition, November 2014

**Printed in
THE UNITED STATES of AMERICA**

FOR MY FRIENDS

(those I know personally, those I have had the pleasure

of meeting, and those I haven't met yet)

who have experienced struggle

with the physical and psychological issues

of diet, weight, health, and happiness,

I dedicate this book to you.

There is an easy way to lasting radiance.

YOU are perfect.

If I can do it,

YOU CAN DO IT!

love,
TARA

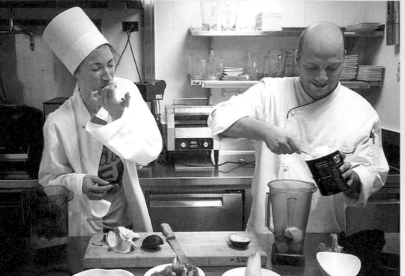
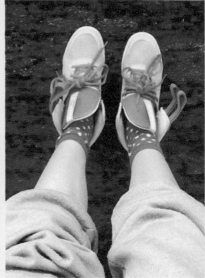
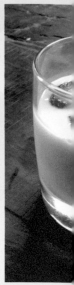
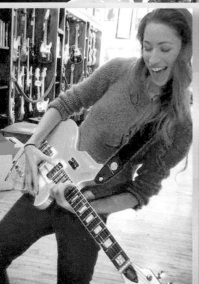
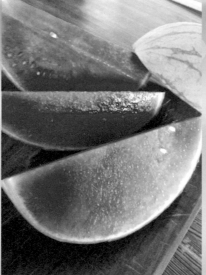
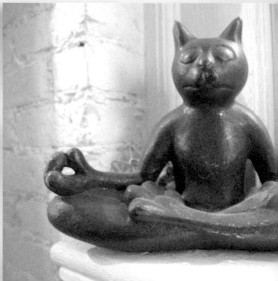
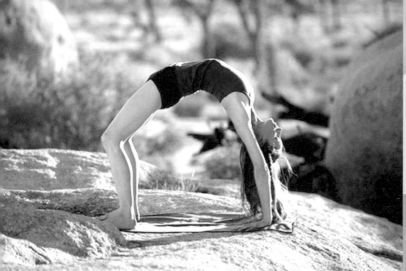
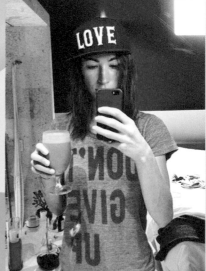
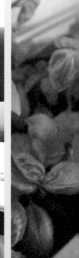

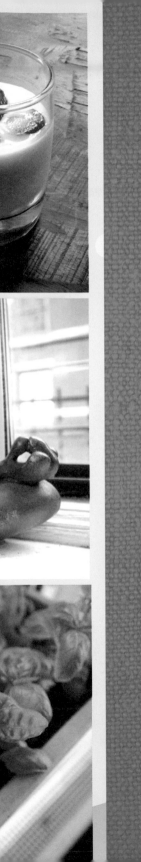

contents

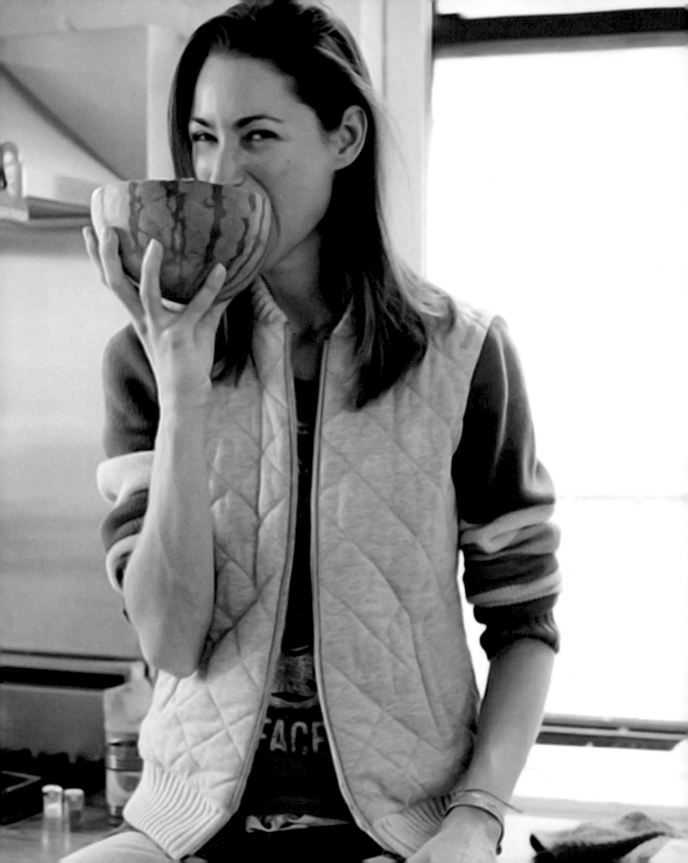

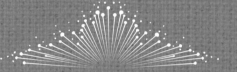

foreword
by mark hyman, M.D.

THere is only one way to health. your way!
I often say to my patients that there is no better book on your health than the book of your own body. Read it, listen to it, tune in to it, cultivate a relationship with it, notice what makes it feel great, and notice what makes it feel not so great. It will be the best book you ever read. In this honest, transparent, intimate invitation to ourselves,

Make Your Own Rules Diet, Tara Stiles encourages us all to read the book of our own body and our own life, and see what it has to say. Left aside are the dogma, dictums, rules, prescriptions, and ideas that often get in the way of completely connecting with what our own body and soul require to thrive. Each of us is different. And yet we all require special care and feeding that is essential for being a vibrant human.

It is astonishing that most of us have never learned the simple rules that work for us, never learned how to feed and care for our one precious human body and soul. We never learned how to reset, renew, rebalance, and restore our inner compass—a compass that will naturally guide us to what to eat, how much to rest, how to move, how to love, and how to be happy. What would it take for each of us to stop, listen, and discover how to deeply nourish ourselves?

There are simple practices and life skills that are required to thrive and live the life we dream. These are what make everything else possible and connect us to what's important. These practices allow us to manifest health, meaningful work, easeful play, family, love, community, connection, and more.

In *Make Your Own Rules Diet,* three life skills—how to move our bodies, calm our minds, and nourish ourselves—are made exceedingly simple, accessible, and even exciting. All you need is a yoga mat, a cushion, and a kitchen. With

Tara's guidance and love, it feels fun and easy and unavoidable to do the right thing. No judgment, no fixing, no worrying, no stressing, no goal, no right way. Just a playful encouragement to try a few things: flowing through some simple yoga poses to unwind the stuck places in our bodies; sitting still for once and listening in mediation; and making friends with your kitchen, the grocery store, and your own capacity to nourish yourself with simple, real food.

Think of the *Make Your Own Rules Diet* as the love diet—a way to love yourself no matter what. It will help you build a simple path to healing that you can come back to over and over again when life takes you down a dark alley or side street. Stress finds us. Life tumbles us around and sometimes knocks us off our feet. But Tara shows us how to get back to home base, to find our way back to balance. And it ain't that hard or mysterious. When you make a wrong turn driving your car, your GPS doesn't say, "Hey, you stupid idiot, why did you go that way? I told you where to go. Are you a moron or something?" No, it gently reminds you to turn back to where you are going at the next possible opportunity in a loving, kind voice. That is what Tara has given us, a GPS for our bodies, minds, and souls; and in a kind, loving way she shows us how to get back to where we want to be in life. Thank you, Tara, you rocked it!

MARK HYMAN, M.D.

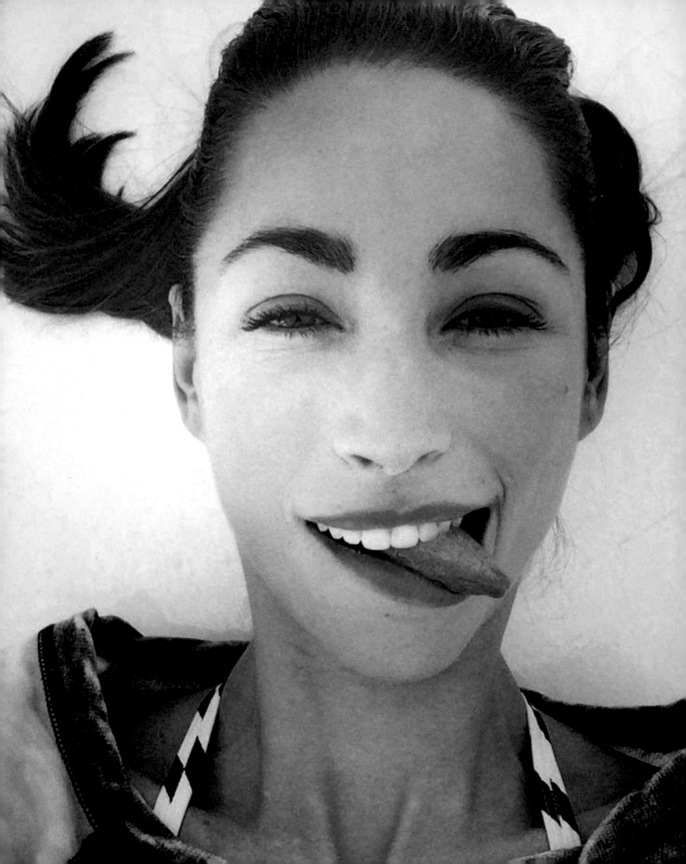

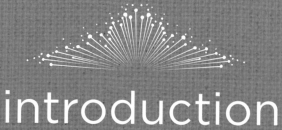

introduction

Make your own rules. Break your own rules. Except when it comes to traffic lights; you'll want to pay attention to those.

Who made the rules that govern our lives, and why are we following them? When you put yourself in the position of a follower, you're at the back of a long line, waiting for a golden ticket that is bound to be counterfeit. Most of the time you end up empty-handed and more frustrated than when you stepped in line. Sound familiar? We've all signed up for diets, plans, systems, and products that promised to change our bodies, minds, and lives for the better, but they almost always end up collecting dust in a corner, and we end up in a loop of continuously searching for the next fix.

Sure, there is value in experimenting and finding inspiration. But when following someone else's rules leads us further away from ourselves, we start swimming in dangerous territory. We chase the external and grasp at the next best thing that never lives up to its promise. And worse yet, we begin to think of ourselves as failures. We messed up that diet. We dropped the ball on that big plan. We weren't successful with that system. But there's a very important secret here: We've never failed ourselves. We've only proven again and again that other people's rules, other people's footsteps, simply belong to other people!

Whether the expectations, pressures, and judgments come from someone else or from within, we too often feel bad about ourselves and begin to shut down. We start life full of zest, inspiration, and big open ideas about what we would like to do and experience. But along the way we find ways to block ourselves from our dreams and desires. We build walls, form bubbles, and make rules that hold us back from living healthy, happy, and radiant lives.

All the frustration, pain, and guilt that come along with trying to live in a predetermined manner lead to an unhealthy life. We get tense. We get scared. We run out of room to breathe, feel, think, and be ourselves. We get backed into a corner. What I've found—in my own life and the lives of thousands of people I've worked with as the founder of Strala—is that the key to creating a healthy life starts with stepping out of that corner and creating an authentic feeling of space.

We all feel great when we have space for ourselves. Room to breathe, feel, think, and exist. When we lack that space, we often (unknowingly) form destructive habits to provide the temporary illusion of it. We can't escape our need for space, but we can change how we create and sustain room for ourselves so we can live happy, healthy lives. And that's what this book is all about—finding your space.

If you think about it, you'll see that you are a space maker. Every big inhale you take creates room inside your body and mind. The deeper you breathe, the more space opens up.

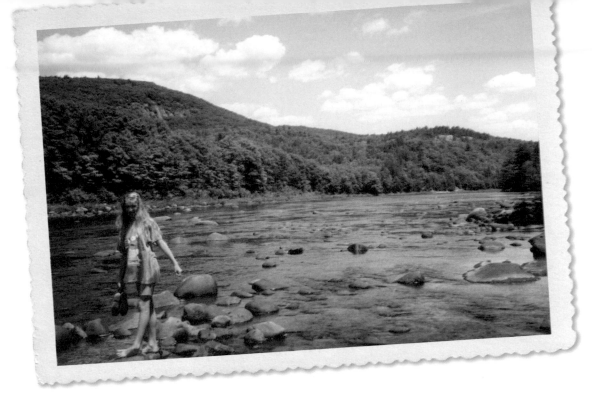

When I was a little kid, I would go out to the woods and sit, close my eyes, and breathe. I loved this time by myself and felt superconnected to the earth and my place on it. This time alone fueled my creativity and inspiration. I saw lots of colors all around that appeared to me to be the universe dancing. They were brighter than neon, in all shades and vibrancies. It was like having my own personal show from the universe every time I decided to sit and breathe.

When I created space for myself, I was able to enjoy nature's beauty and get some inspirational messages that seemed to be coming, simultaneously, from deep inside and all around me. The more space I had, the more room there was for my intuition and creativity to thrive. And this is true for all of us. With space, stress levels go down. Feeling great goes up. The more space you have, the better you start to feel and the more you'll want to continue the great feeling. The more space you have, the more aware you will be about what your body and mind need in order to feel good. The practices in this book will help rewire your brain so you intuitively know what will make you feel good and what will make you ill. And after living this way for a while, you will actually want to treat yourself well, eat better, and be more mindful and kinder to yourself. Great stuff begins right now and right inside you.

MAKE YOUR OWN RULES JOURNEY

So now let's go on a space-making journey together. We'll cast aside the rules that other people have laid out; you'll learn how to tap into your intuition to create rules that work for you. And because this is all about you, you're in charge. I'll simply be your guide. I'll keep you safe, give you support and love, and pull you up when you need it. I'll share my personal stories of ups and downs and finding ease; plus I'll give you inspiration from friends who have gone through a lot and come out in line with their intuition. I know you'll be inspired and excited to take your own journey inward and make your own rules.

The work you are about to do is all about getting in touch with yourself. You will become sensitive to what you need in the moment because you'll be able to tap into your intuition. This connection to yourself is so powerful that it will guide you exactly where you want to go. And that's what makes this program different. It's not about cutting calories, working out all the time, or worrying about everything. It's about knowing yourself, so you can get a ridiculously strong, gorgeous body from the inside out. You will make space in yourself and gain a clear, calm, and focused mind full of creativity, plus the ability to enjoy life without getting dragged down by stress and tension. Most important, you'll gain access to your energy, your power, and your potential. I know I am making big promises to you, but I can do this because I've seen the results with loads of people who follow these practices. I'm so excited for you!

The plan is simple and effective, and it focuses on three areas—the mat, the cushion, and the kitchen. I'll walk you through the benefits of yoga, meditation, and making your own meals while stressing the importance of staying true to who you are and what you need. I'll teach you how to make your own rules and set your own goals. Since this is your path, with your rules, you'll be able to create it in a way that you love. But don't worry; I won't leave you without practical tools and techniques. You'll find multiple yoga routines, meditation practices, and oodles of simple, delicious recipes.

At the end of the book, you'll find two day-by-day programs that you can use if you want to. There's the 7 Days to Radiate Kick Start and a 30-Day Real-Deal Transformation

Plan. If you follow these, I promise you'll feel amazing. You'll be calm, connected, and happy. But if you don't want to go exactly by these plans, don't! Remember, it's all about you. Feel free to create your own transformation plan, picking and choosing from what's in the book—or from what you have learned in other books or in your other experiences. Make your own rules!

I've personally been down the road to being connected, disconnected, and back home to being reconnected. And believe me: there is no place like home! This isn't another quick fix or fad. This is the real road back to you living above and beyond your ideal health, energy levels, and vibrancy.

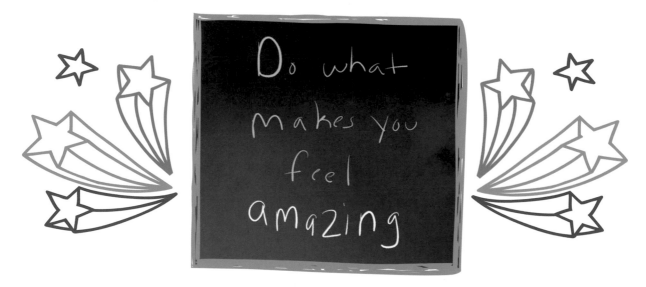

Do what makes you feel amazing

This philosophy and way of living isn't just another book to write to fill my time. It's the fuel to my fire and the core of what connects me to my purpose on the planet. This is *it,* my friends. This message is so powerful and transformative that I can't imagine spending my time cultivating or delivering anything else. I see so many people struggling with weight, energy, body image, anger, and stress issues, and it hurts my heart because I know it is unnecessary. They just need to make the space for themselves. They need to learn to live with ease and find the joy in who they are. This is my wish for all of them—and for you! There's great stuff waiting for you, so let's get started!

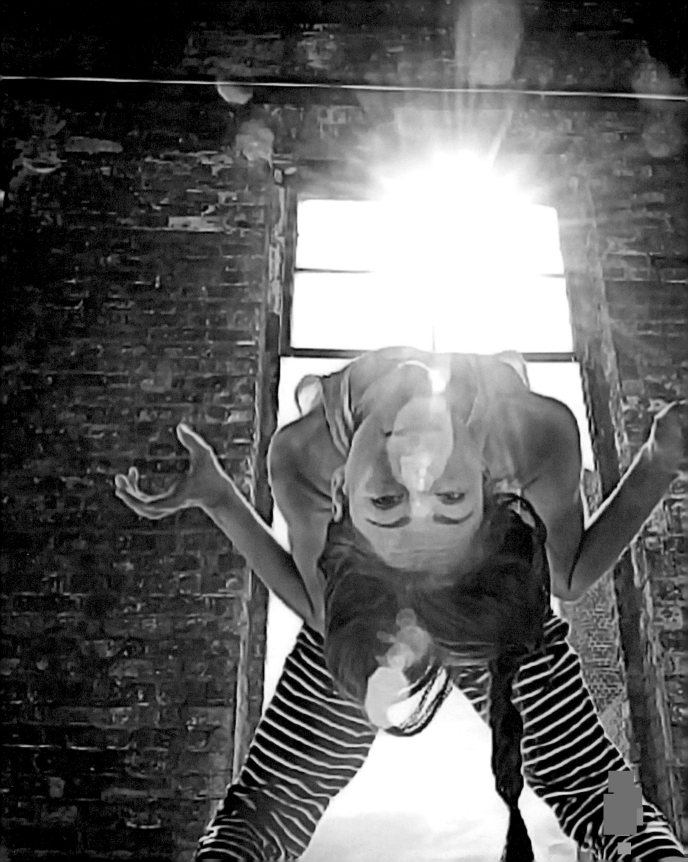

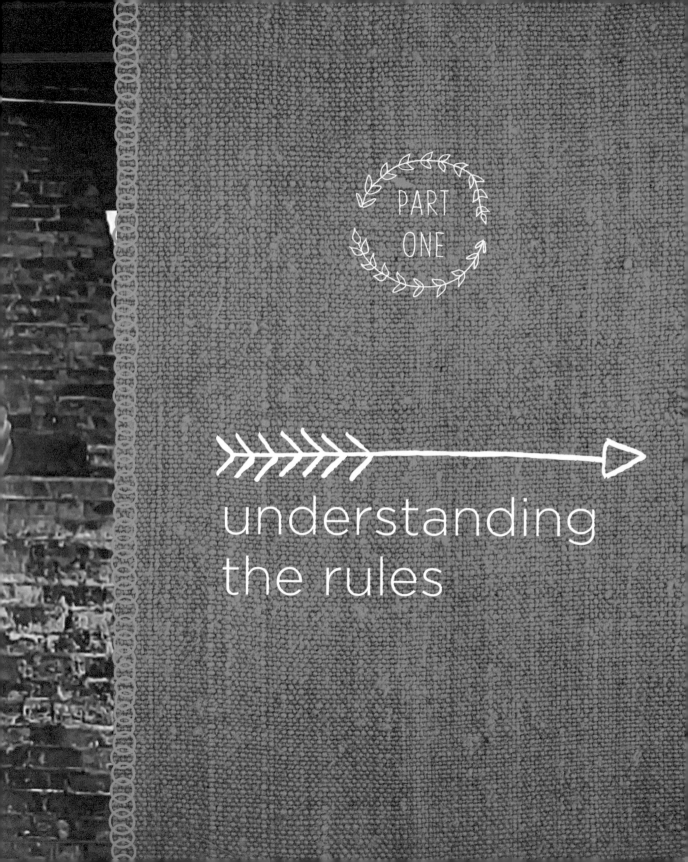

PART
ONE

understanding
the rules

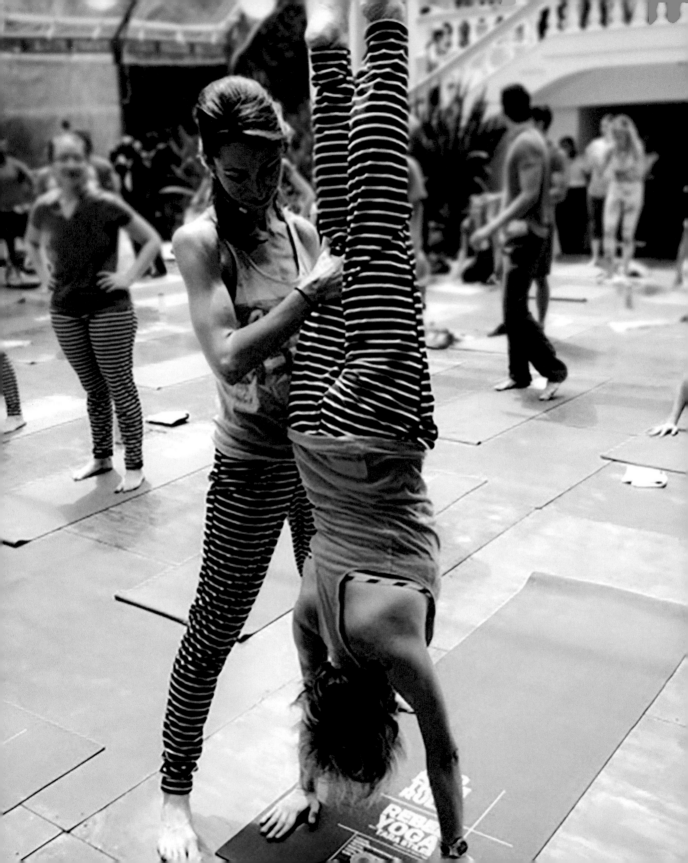

the rules
of the world

Many of us grow up learning that things are supposed to be hard. School, sports, relationships, careers, and family take hard work. Life is tough, but if you work harder than everyone else, you'll have a shot at success. You have to be tough to beat your competition. You have to be tense in order to prove how hard you're working. If you relax, you'll be passed up, forgotten, and never achieve your goals. No pain, no gain. Sound familiar?

These rules have worked their way into every aspect of our lives. We become proud of how much we can take on and how much we can accomplish, and we fail to recognize the damage we are causing in the meantime. Living by these rules makes us desensitized to what we truly need and what will truly make us happy.

In our day-to-day lives, we are often at war with ourselves internally and in conflict with many things that come our way. How we feel on the inside affects how we feel about everything around us. When we are desensitized, anxious, tense, and frustrated, the slightest slip from how we expect things to go in our day can throw us way off. We rely on our house of cards to hold up to life's twists and turns. If we are calm, grounded, centered, and sensitized, it doesn't shake us much when something doesn't quite go our way. When we are sensitized, we have the space to calmly focus and do what we need to do about the situation without anxiety and stress taking over.

When we lose touch with ourselves, we begin to shut down and search for space and pleasure wherever we can find it: sugars, fats, caffeine, fast and fried food—pick your vice—become our friends that help stuff down the tension we feel and give us some temporary peace. Unfortunately, our bad-news friends don't have good intentions. They are designed to feed into a cycle of tension and pleasure and trap us under the results of poor habits: an imbalanced life, weight gain, sickness, and feeling down about ourselves.

Often, instead of living out our dreams, reaching our goals, and enjoying life, we get stuck in gaining tension, frustration, and unease, which manifests in agitated views about our bodies and minds. We find ways to punish and reward ourselves and form all sorts of self-abusing behaviors, from destructive thought patterns to imbalanced and unhealthy relationships with food, ourselves, and the people in our lives. Our intuition can't help us when we drift so far away from it. We have to be connected in order to navigate. When we are able to find ease in our lives, we can begin to dissolve the tension and get right back on the path to intuition lane, which takes us directly to our most fantastic selves.

FOOD AND HEALTH

When you think about what being desensitized means in terms of our health and our relationships with food, it's really scary. Eating is supposed to be one of life's greatest pleasures. We eat for social and family gatherings. We eat as a community. We eat with friends and lovers, and by ourselves. We eat for fuel, and we eat for fun. We eat to celebrate. We eat when it's mealtime. We eat several times a day, every day.

When we're kids, we enjoy food without worry or guilt. We eat when we're hungry. We love the feeling of tasting something yummy. We love the feeling of being satisfied after a great meal. We take that energy and play. When we need more fuel, we look for something delicious to eat.

But soon enough the rules of society make us switch from enjoyment- and feeling-based eating to analytical and worry-based calorie counting. Our new-thinking brains squash all the fun and joy out of the experience of food, and soon we're sucked into a box of restraint and anxiety. Something yummy transforms into something that shouldn't be eaten or, simply, a whole lot of calories. The feeling of being satisfied after a great meal becomes laced with guilt and remorse. We use the energy to worry and stress instead of play. When we do play, we analyze that, too. We choose our play based on how many calories we can burn. Play turns into a frustrated, anxiety-based, calorie-burning task. We no longer enjoy eating, and we no longer enjoy play.

When we stop trusting how we feel and start looking at the numbers of calories in and calories burned, we are laying down some pretty strict rules for ourselves that don't add up. The results we get are never as great as our plans. If our misadventures in calorie counting and burning were subject to the same scrutiny as our financial lives, we'd be in some serious trouble with audits, back payments, and loads of fines.

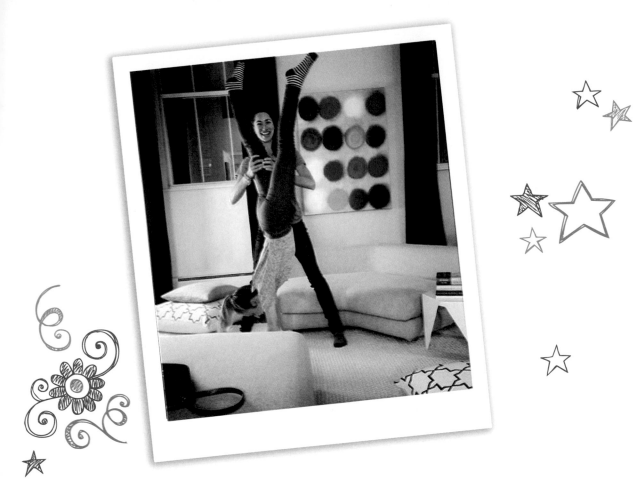

This emphasis on calorie counting and burning desensitizes us even more and reinforces the misconception that we should be analyzing instead of feeling. We move further from our intuition and find ourselves wrestling with a broken pattern of punishment and reward: we cut calories because we feel bad, we work out, we feel proud, we reward ourselves with food; then we feel bad and start all over.

Punishment and reward is a cycle that we fall into easily in our busy lives—and not just with eating. Work life is hard. Family life is consuming. Schedules are jam-packed. We have no space for ourselves. We have no opportunity during our busy days to actually feel. Soon enough we lose the desire to feel. It's easier to go on autopilot, stuff down our emotions, and take things on rather than take things in. We pile on the weight, responsibility, and baggage, and have no outlet to free ourselves.

LOSING YOURSELF

When it comes to getting healthy, not only do we have to worry about the punishment-and-reward cycle desensitizing us; we also have to deal with problems in our food supply, societal pressures, and events that lead us away from ourselves. Natural foods are often modified from their original forms and presented to us with the intent to exploit our feelings of failure and disappointment. Fake sugars, processed salts, chemicals, colors, and smells trick our minds into believing that our problems will be solved if we down a bag of Doritos, clean out a pint of Ben & Jerry's, or hit the drive-through on the way home from a stressful day.

Teams of highly paid consultants decide how best to deceive us into consuming the most junk food in the largest quantities to keep us addicted. It's comforting and scary to know that much of the food nonsense isn't our fault; it's what is put in the food and marketed to us. Knowing what kinds of junk items are available and knowing what they do to us when we consume them regularly is valuable information and fuel for us to eat more naturally so we can feel better.

We all know by now to some degree or another, depending on how much Googling we do and how many local farmers and food industry insiders are in our inner circle, that the food industry has evolved to make us fat, get us sick, and give us life-ending diseases. "Obesity is such that this generation of children could be the first basically in the history of the United States to live less healthful and shorter lives than their parents," said Dr. David S. Ludwig, director of the obesity program at Boston Children's Hospital, in a *New York Times* article. Shorter lives are not the only risk. Quality of life is affected as well. Type 2 diabetes, heart disease, kidney failure, and cancer are likely to affect people at younger and younger ages.

Aside from the messed-up stuff happening with our actual food supply, we deal with insane amounts of pressure from advertisements and the media. Photoshopped images we see in magazines are a superdistorted version of reality that tries to fool us into believing we need to change everything about ourselves in an attempt to fit into an unreal image. We lose sight of the fact that we actually are beautiful and perfectly unique. We lose sight of the fact that we are born to be individually awesome, not to fit into an artificially generated mold that actually looks like no human alive. Our digital age can warp our body image easily if we let it. We have to actively work to stay centered and true to who we are and constantly build our self-esteem.

Events in our lives occur that pull us off balance and away from our intuition. Traumatic experiences and social pressures of all sorts swing us way off course. We all go through tough times in our lives. It's how we survive and thrive that makes the difference. Not-so-fun things are going to happen. We have to build the strength to remember that when we come back to center, we come back to the path of feeling happy and grounded, and back to the path of sustainable health and happiness. You are worth so much in this life. Don't ever forget it.

And let's not forget one of the biggest intuition killers . . .

TIME FOR A BREAKUP

Diets are the worst thing you can do if you're looking to get back to a healthy life. They are fundamentally designed to be cheated on, broken up with, and crawled back to with desperation. They tell us that we aren't good enough, don't know enough, and aren't equipped with the skills we need to be healthy and happy and to feel great in our ideal bodies. Diets tell us we are broken. Diets lure us in with deceptive promises of external results while attempting to control our every move. Diets teach us to hold our breath, to grin and bear it. Diets tell us, "If it were easy to be healthy and have a great body, everyone would." Diets tell us we have to go through them to get to ourselves. Diets teach us to hate ourselves, and they show us many ways to practice aggression and tension toward ourselves.

Diets are no good for us. They don't work, and they waste our time while leading us further away from our ideal selves. If a diet were a person that we were involved with, hopefully our close friends would stage an intervention and tell us to break up and end the cycle of abuse for good.

make your own rules diet

We all know that diets don't work. Diet fads are so popular because we try, we fail, we get desperate, and we jump on the next one. We don't stop to consider that the failure might not be our own. And there is always a next one. Our dependence on diets could be the reason 70 percent of the population is set to be obese by 2022. Whoa . . . now that's heavy!

Looking outward for fear-based motivation and diet rules might at best help you temporarily drop a few pounds. But in no way will looking outward for satisfaction or direction ever get you lasting health, sustainable happiness, and the body shape and mental clarity you've been looking for. You might have been searching a long time for the answers, and maybe you forgot to dive into the source, where the answers are waiting for you to discover them: right within you!

Whether too heavy or too thin, the external result is hardly the root of the problem. An unhealthy relationship with food takes on many forms: eating disorders, emotional eating and restricting, overly healthy control behaviors, exercise addiction, and diet obsession—the list is endless. Every person is unique and every relationship is unique. Our only hope for lifelong health begins in understanding that it's not about the food and it's not about the diet. It's about you and how you feel. It's about getting connected.

MY STORY:
FALLING OFF BALANCE . . . WAY OFF

For me, like many of us, losing track of myself was a slow process. I spent my childhood eating pretty naturally, fresh from the garden and the farm in Illinois where I grew up. I ate when I was hungry, and I ate things that fueled my body and made me feel good.

I had loads of energy. I'd run around and play all day and sleep well through the night. I danced after school until late and had enough energy to feel great through all of it. My mind was clear and sharp. Focusing on schoolwork was easy, and there was plenty of space for daydreams and wondering about the world and where I would be in it through my years. I had no idea what a craving was besides being hungry. I ate when I was hungry and stopped when I was full.

As a teenager, I started dancing in a conservatory program in Chicago. I was excited but also a little terrified to leave my big-fish-small-pond situation for a large sea of talented dancers from around the world. I loved the challenge, opportunity, and inspiration, and I threw myself in headfirst. After a few weeks in the program, I was living a schedule of wake up, go to dance class, go to rehearsal, sleep, wake up, and so on—nonstop. One night I wandered my tired body back to my dorm room, so excited to crash, only to discover a huge party happening in my room. I was exhausted and wanted to tuck myself in for the night, but seeing that I was overruled by ragers and finding no other option, I took a plastic cup of whatever was handed to me and started sipping a mystery drink. I figured I would just wait it out.

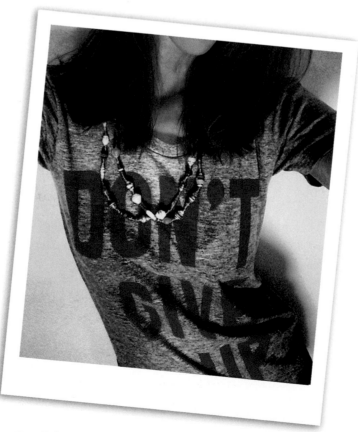

The next thing I remember, there was a naked man on top of me in a room that wasn't my own. I was confused, petrified, and frozen. I had no idea what had happened. The door was closed, and no one else was in the room. I tried to play it cool and get out of there without screaming. I managed to get out and ran back to my room, collapsing to the floor, huddling into a ball, and sobbing uncontrollably. My roommate eventually found me. I told her what happened, and she did her best to comfort me.

Every ounce of my intuition vanished in that moment like a lightning bolt. During the moments, days, weeks, and months that passed, I transformed into a zombie. I became extremely withdrawn, stopped eating, and began isolating myself as much as possible. I didn't report anything because I didn't know what had actually happened. I didn't know anything except I felt like disappearing.

I composed a complex routine that kept me in isolation as much as possible. I woke up hours earlier than my roommate, tiptoed out of the room, went for a run, and stayed away from people until dance classes began. I went off on my own during meal breaks to minimize the chance of interacting with anyone and then returned to rehearsal as though nothing were wrong.

I became more and more isolated, and I was losing more and more weight. I hated eating because it made me feel good, and I didn't want to feel anything. Empty felt okay. I took a part-time job in the conservatory's cafeteria as a baker so I could lie about when and what I ate. It also allowed me to hide during normal mealtimes. Controlling my body and restricting my food became something I could control. The act of controlling gave me something to do and something that I could be in charge of. Control was the root of my problem. I could not control what had happened to me, so I tried to make up for it. My external world was chaotic, intense, and scary. I was spinning out of control, and I was completely desensitized.

From the outside it must have looked as if I were developing anorexia because of the physical and mental stress that is common among young dancers. I was so afraid of being judged as a typical dancer with an eating disorder that I withdrew even more. I was too afraid to talk to anyone about what had or hadn't happened.

To make matters even more intense, I saw the guy almost every day. He was the boyfriend of an older dancer in the program. He would come to pick her up and drop her off. I froze and tried to act normal anytime I saw him. The last thing I wanted to do was confront what had happened or feel what was actually going on inside me.

My actions began to destroy my body like a violent tornado. It whipped through me, leaving nothing but wreckage and pieces of a once happy, lively girl. My bones started protruding. My ribs started poking out in the front and then through my back. My strength was fading, and my focus and concentration drifted. My life became fuzzy and strange. I felt things slipping away. I noticed people talking about how thin I had become, and I felt judged and misunderstood. I heard snickers and whispers wherever I went.

Even worse, my behaviors affected others. Some of the aspiring dancers who looked up to me started to starve themselves to be like me—a side effect that was heartbreaking. I didn't have the strength or confidence to help the girls or myself in those moments. Witnessing their self-abuse was torture. A wall of guilt and shame went up around me. I hated that I had influence and that my self-abuse seemed like a good idea to copy. I was constantly embarrassed and hiding. I hated that people thought I was manipulating my body in order to achieve a skinny look. I was the only one who knew about my secret need for control, and I hated myself for behaving this way.

Life just kept going on like this until one day when I was on my way to a performance. As I walked down an empty hallway, I saw my ballet teacher, who was actually pivotal in guiding me toward pursuing yoga, walking toward me. My heart sank. There was no one around, and I knew he was going to confront me. There was no escape. My hands felt sweaty, and I was shaking. I braced myself to be judged, and then something life changing happened.

He stopped me, touched my arm with kindness, and gently told me that if I didn't nourish myself, my body would eat itself and there would be nothing left. I was so embarrassed and mumbled something about how busy I was, promising that I would make time to take care of myself. He saw right through me and knew

I understood his message. I was so ashamed that I didn't have the courage to tell him why I had been destroying myself. His message hit me, softened me, and I decided to make a change. I was lucky.

Soon after that moment of grace and kindness, I moved out of the dorm and into an apartment with roommates. I reintroduced myself to food, taking care of myself, and healing. I found ways to regain control of my life and to feel safe in my own skin and in my surroundings. I relearned what it felt like to feel, and I practiced feeling my way through life again. I found yoga classes and healing centers, and I allowed the process to begin.

The road to recovery wasn't fast and it wasn't straight, but it was steady and it worked. Allowing myself to feel again helped me. Allowing myself to become sensitized through dance, yoga, meditation, and long walks in nature helped me. Telling this story to a few close friends at the time helped me. And now, sharing this story with you helps me close the loop and open the healing process to anyone who has gone through or experienced any kind of trauma that leads directly to desensitization and self-destruction. There is a way back to you, and trust me—if I can do it, you can do it.

IT DOESN'T HAVE TO BE PAINFUL

It's pretty obvious that the folks who have been laying out the optimal health and diet rules over the years have gotten it way wrong, and we've paid the price big-time. It's been criminal, and it has gone without punishment. Even worse, we continue to look to the diet makers, the nutritionists, and the companies that call themselves food providers for answers. We empower others to control us. We continue to buy the products, supplements, and meal plans. We buy into whatever has the biggest promise. We lose our sense of self, along with our health. We have become the biggest losers of our health. So it's time to change! It's time to get to know what you really need, to get to know yourself.

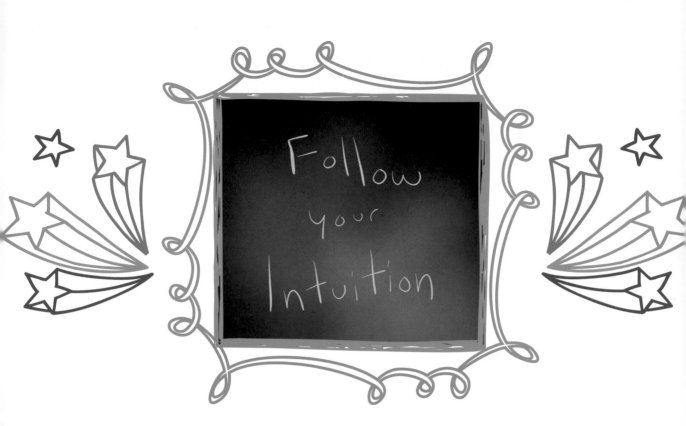

Getting intuitive will be the most rewarding, life-changing decision you ever make. The moment you decide to put other people's rules aside and shift into the mode of intuition and self-discovery is the moment you take your power back. It only gets better from here.

Making your own rules is a practice of feeling your way into every part of you. Traditional diets, exercise plans, and how we've been shown to deal with pretty much everything in life has taught us how to disconnect and turn off intuition like a switch. No pain, no gain. Hold your breath. Push through the discomfort. It's not supposed to be easy if you want to get anywhere. Of course, we already know these things don't work. How could they? Turning off our feelings, disconnecting from ourselves, doesn't work *for* us. It works *against* us.

So let's learn how to breathe through every feeling and dive deeper into every aspect that makes up you. We'll enjoy the process of cultivating a healthy and strong body, a calm and focused mind, and a spectacularly capable life. You're going to go inside, get intuitive, get excited, and get inspired, and the best part is, you're going to have a ton of fun! Being you is fun! Trying to be all those other people and follow their rules is a big energy drain. Get ready to step out of the followers' line. Get ready to not just reach your goals but to blow past them. Anything is possible when you are feeling your way into you.

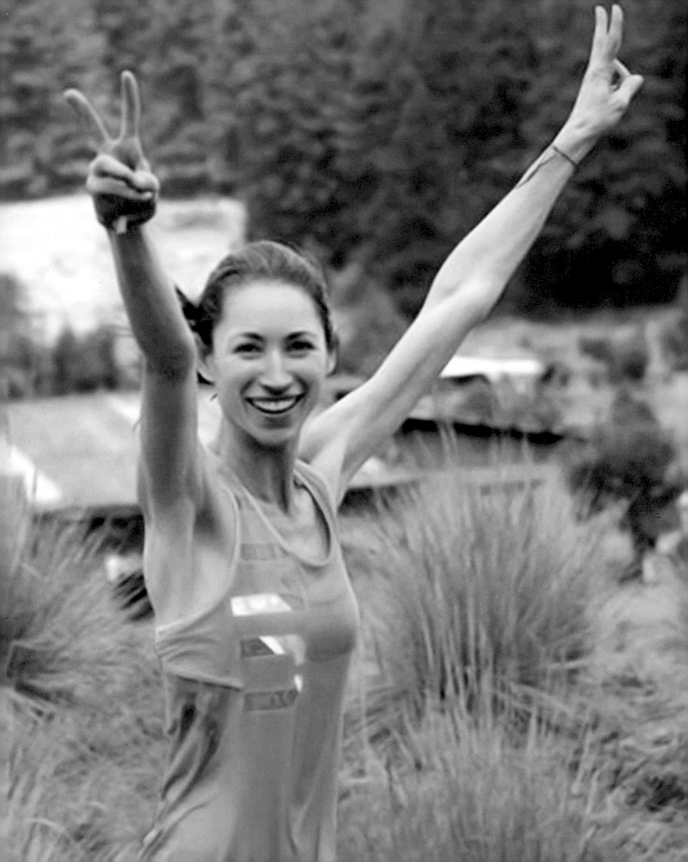

the rules of you

I've been super into nature since I was a kid. I loved to disappear into the woods for hours, talk to the animals, and soak up the inspiration of who and what we are. We aren't so separate from the land and the animals if you really think about it. We are literally made up of the same stuff as the land and the stars. And we can learn a lot from observing nature. Nature has a way of correcting itself, adjusting, and making its own rules, without asking permission or second-guessing. When it's time to rain, it rains. When it's time for the clouds to part, they part. The sky doesn't have a multistep self-help process about how to deal with that pesky rain, wind, and snow; it all simply works together in harmony. Even with aggressive storms and natural disasters, our planet is merely correcting an imbalance.

Nature has many things figured out. It goes with the flow, follows its instincts, uses what it needs, leaves what it doesn't, recycles each season, and begins each day renewed. Plants and trees and animals don't seem to have body issues, eating disorders, or social complexes. They don't subscribe to crash diets and rigorous fitness plans. It would be funny to see an animal check herself out in a mirror with anything other than curiosity. Animals don't pinch their fat, suck in their bellies, step on scales, binge, purge, overexercise, or take diet pills in attempts to reach their ideal weight. It doesn't cross their minds because how they live creates and renews their ideal weight and health in every moment. They make their own rules, they feel into themselves, they follow their intuition, and they seem to have it figured out.

When we allow ourselves to operate like the animals in nature—as living, breathing, interconnected organisms that allow feeling to take the lead—we will be in balance, have radiantly healthy bodies and calm, focused minds, and enjoy living in our ideal bodies.

Luckily we can cultivate the calm, centered, and intuitive way of living. It just takes practice. We can train ourselves to become peaceful soldiers, navigating our lives with grace and ease, radiating space and calm out into the world, and helping others to do the same in the process. It's all about living with ease, which for many of us seems unnatural—definitely not easy.

To learn to live with ease, we have to get back in touch with ourselves. We have to recognize our habits and reactions—the wiring that guides how we handle stress in our lives. While scientists used to believe that the mind was set in adulthood—that we couldn't change how we act, what emotions come up, and so on—we have since learned that the mind is constantly changing. And we can reprogram it so we react in healthy ways and have healthy desires. We can change our wiring by changing our actions. What we are born with isn't what we have to live with. This goes for all sorts of things—from diseases to stress management.

There
is
always
Movement
in
Balance

GETTING SENSITIZED

Getting sensitized is the secret to making your own rules and living a life of ease. When you are sensitized, you are living in feeling mode, instead of thinking and worrying mode. Sure, you still have reason and rational thought, but you aren't ruled by your anxieties or fears anymore. You'll cultivate the ability to exercise choice instead of being tossed around on an emotional roller coaster. With practice you'll begin to muster the courage to believe in and respond to what you feel. And the more you trust and act on your feelings, the easier it gets. You get what you practice, so you might as well practice something that leads you directly to the greatness that exists right inside, waiting for you to discover it.

You are your own best laboratory. You can choose to explore how you are when tension arrives in your life. You can choose to move toward actions that fuel and create more tension, or you can move toward actions that allow tension to be released from your body and mind. When you practice being tense, your body and mind build armor against you and create a big divide between you and your optimal healthy self. When you practice being tense, over time you get

further and further away from your intuition. When you practice being tense, you can't feel when your body and mind are in crisis mode until it's too late. You must choose to practice ease. When you practice living with ease, your body's natural relaxation response ignites and the mind–body connection has space to do great things for you. You don't have to try to stop your self-destructive behaviors.

At first, living with ease has to be a conscious choice, but soon enough the mind–body connection takes over, and your mind wants to keep it going—the more you practice living with ease, the easier it becomes. You actually want to eat things that make you feel great. You actually want to make time for self-care. You actually want to practice yoga and meditation daily. You actually want to eat more fruits and vegetables. Living healthy becomes not a chore or something you feel you should be doing; it becomes something you look forward to, something that feels natural, and something you create a lifestyle around.

ELISE'S TENSE-TO-EASE TRANSFORMATION

Elise is a 20-year-old college student who has struggled with body and anxiety issues and was hospitalized for an eating disorder. After only one week of practicing Strala, where we focus on ease instead of poses, she spontaneously recognized in class one day that she had dropped all her unhealthy and disordered tendencies without even focusing on trying to change. She stopped restricting and counting calories and noticed she was actually enjoying cooking for herself and eating healthy foods. Essentially, she had escalated her recovery process a thousand times over by shifting into ease over analysis. After several months of practice, Elise shifted from being disconnected to being sensitized by simply paying attention to how she feels instead of pushing aside her intuition. Her result was an instant connection to herself, where she felt no need for her past destructive behaviors.

THERE IS NOTHING WRONG WITH YOU

The first step to getting back in tune with yourself so you can live with ease seems somewhat basic, but it is often the biggest stumbling block that people come across. I'm talking about an underlying belief that many people have about themselves: they're not good enough. So let's get one thing out in the open right away. There is nothing wrong with you. You aren't broken. You don't need to be fixed. Go ahead and take it in. We've all experienced moments of just feeling awesome, like anything is possible. Maybe when you were five, you flew around the house like Wonder Woman and exclaimed, "I'm awesome!" Or maybe there was a moment of fierce accomplishment when you finished something tough, such as running a marathon or closing a big deal at work, and you felt invincible. Maybe you've experienced an amazing moment in meditation where you felt calm, connected, and exactly on the right path. I'm sure many of these moments have happened to you, but for some reason, they're fleeting. We forget them. We forget our intuition, and we become insecure and worried—and then we develop this wacky idea that we're broken. My favorite thing to do when I meet with people in person who are worried about being broken is to place my hand on their head, smile really big, and say, "Demons out!" And then we hug. It's important. You are perfect, just like the trees, just like the wind, just like the stars. You might need a moment to take this in, so here's a quick practice you can do that will help start to change any ill-conceived perceptions you may have about yourself. Try it now.

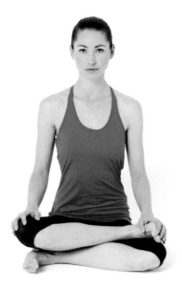

Sit however you can be comfortable. You can be on a chair, in bed, or on the floor. If you are on a chair, even your body so both feet are on the floor or your legs are folded up cross-legged on your chair. The main thing is to be comfortable; it's not about sitting like your idea of a perfect meditation statue. If you are on the floor, try sitting cross-legged or on your heels. Sit up tall. Relax your head, neck, and shoulders. Rest your hands on your thighs. Relax your face. Relax your whole body. Now take a giant, deep breath in. Hold it for a moment. Feel yourself be full, spacious, and content. Now gently let all the air out. Keep breathing easily for a few moments, enjoying the space inside you. Then say either in your mind or out loud, "There is nothing wrong with me. I have room to breathe."

Incorporate this practice into your daily routine. Whether you are in an already-feeling-awesome state or far from it, this simple habit will bring you back to calm, connected, and remembering how great you really are.

This small meditation can give you just the little bit of encouragement you need to start on your path to listening to your intuition—and you can use it any-time you start to doubt yourself along your journey. Remember, when we stray from our intuition, we get tossed in the sea of insecurities. We are programmed to believe we are supposed to look like photos of other people, who, for the most part, don't look like their photos in real life! We are tricked into believing we should log a certain number on the scale and stay at that number for eternity without fluctuation. We believe that we should fit into a certain dress size that has nothing to do with how our body is right now.

Part of taking your own walk and making your own rules is that you start where you are—that's right where you need to be. You have to like where you are in order to like where you are going. The answers you need along the way are the only place that your answers could ever be: inside you! The reality is that your ideal self is completely attainable, and the process will be an adventure. There is no need to grin and bear it. There will be no wrinkled-up-face poses in the process. Together we will find the ease through the simple and the challenging. You'll learn how to like yourself, and you'll learn how to enjoy being you through the journey of becoming intuitive. You'll make your own rules and love it.

THINGS TO REMEMBER

As you're beginning your journey to a life of ease, there are a few things that you should keep in mind. If you can remember to do these basic things, you can easily create rules that will help you get back to your best self:

1. Feel. Feeling should be the base for all our rules. Make decisions based on how you feel. Eat based on how you feel.

2. Believe. When you start really feeling into yourself, you have a choice: to believe what you feel or ignore it. Believing in yourself is essential to creating lasting change and a happy life.

3. Move. You need to move. Unfortunately, nobody can be their best self without it. We're animals—we weren't made to just sit around. So, yes, you'll have to move. But remember to do so with ease.

4. **Nourish.** Get in the kitchen and fix up some delicious and healthy meals. It's not that hard, and you really will be able to tell the difference in how you feel. And when you feel great, you want to eat well—so jump on that positive spiral.

5. **Have fun.** I have a policy. If it's not fun, don't do it! Of course there are some things in life we have to do that aren't the most fun, but for the rest of life, we have loads of choices. We choose how we move our bodies, how we think, and what we eat.

FORGET ABOUT THE BURN AND ENJOY YOURSELF

A fitness blogger who once reviewed my RELAX class at Strala said she really enjoyed the class but probably wouldn't put it into her weekly fitness routine because her calorie counter (which she wore on her upper arm during the class) told her she only burned 140 calories. She is very concerned with her calorie-to-burn ratio and is sadly missing all the benefits of feeling. She later came to a STRONG class, one of our classic, sweaty, more athletic classes, and was satisfied with her burn, but I was afraid she was missing the overall benefits of feeling. It just seems too good to be true. Focus on what feels great and you'll end up with more than you desire. It absolutely is true, but the hard part is getting to the feeling, especially when we've gotten so far away from it.

Trusting how you feel and practicing following your intuition is a huge renewable power source that is right inside each of us. We can live our lives without it and follow the rules and path we think we should be on, or we can trust how we feel and live an extraordinary life. And we'll be healthy and radiant in the process. Let's be radiant!

 # PRACTICING HOW

When you are connected to yourself and using your feeling as navigation, you'll never go off course and the results will be beyond fantastic. And thankfully there are tools to help us when we get off track. There are ways to bring us back inward when we get focused on the external. There are steps we can take to come back inside when we spiral out of control. The techniques I outline in this book—meditation, yoga, and cooking—will help you get back in touch with yourself, so you can figure out what rules will serve you well at this point in your life.

These rules will be a moldable, flexible playbook of specific guidelines carefully constructed by your very best possible caregiver and health practitioner: you! The stresses of sticking with someone else's diet plan, fitness plan, ideas, and expectations are completely lifted and tossed out of existence. You are left with clear, wide-open space to begin cultivating a radiantly healthy and happy life from the inside out. The pressure is completely off. You are free to relax and ready to cultivate your most radiant, healthy self. That's why making your own rules works. As long as you're in touch with yourself—as long as you're sensitized—you'll only make rules that will get you to your goals. Exciting stuff!

Anyone I've admired who has invented anything of value, created anything of artistic merit, or changed the world socially has made their own rules. Amelia Earhart soared after men told her she could not. Martin Luther King, Jr., organized nonviolent protests that inspired global change. Joan of Arc led an army to victory to defend her truth—in her teens!

We all have heroes in our daily lives. Mothers, fathers, siblings, children, co-workers, and friends who've improved our lives by going against the stream. My good friend Tao Porchon-Lynch is 96 years young and blazes trails all over the globe, leading yoga classes and reminding people they have the power to accomplish anything.

Our heroes are important to us because they believed in their visions for how life could be when no one else did. They took a giant leap of faith, went against the grain, broke the rules, and left the world a better place.

Sometimes "following the rules" means holding ourselves back. It's easy to fall into habits and stay in our comfort zones. I don't buy the "fear of failure" routine. We can all imagine our own failure. What's more difficult to imagine is our success. It's uncharted, unscripted, and completely unbound. Our success is an adventure waiting for us to go along for the ride.

When you decide to take back control of your life, it's like starting fresh with a clean slate. Your brand-new life starts right now. You get to decide how you want to live, how you want to feel, how you want to act, and how you want to interact with people and your surroundings. A new start is thrilling and a gift you can give to yourself right now. I want to share with you my rules. Feel free to adopt them for yourself, toss in a few of your own that work for you, or make up your own.

1. **Feel.** Feeling is everything. When I am connected to feeling my way around instead of thinking or worrying my way around, my intuition can begin to do its thing.

2. **Breathe deep.** Every inhale creates more space and room inside. Every exhale moves me right into that space. The deeper I breathe, the more space opens up.

3. **Pay attention.** Self-observation is critical for progress. Meditation and yoga provide the outline and the how of feeling; it's up to me to decide to pay attention to how I am, what choices are in my life, and how I want to act and live.

4. **Stay connected.** Regular practice of yoga and meditation: 5 minutes, 10 minutes, an hour every day. Whatever time I have, it's important to make some time every day to get and stay connected to feeling. It's not a one-and-done type thing. It's an everyday practice, habit, and ritual.

5. **Get interested.** The process of living well and exploring is interesting. It's important to take an interest in myself and my surroundings. When

I am interested, things begin to have context and meaning and value. Experience becomes enriched and spherical instead of one-dimensional. The more I stay interested, the more depth my experience takes on.

6. **Take Care.** Taking care of myself is a process and a practice that can be really fun and enjoyable. Long walks, hot baths, nourishing foods, good books, stimulating adventures. Planning self-care time is essential to living well, and I'm worth it!

7. **Hug People.** This is one of my favorite practices. I hug friends, relatives, people at yoga, strangers, flight attendants, and pretty much anyone who will give me an opportunity. A hug is a superwarm, fuzzy, and wholesome way to connect with someone that makes both people feel great. The sense of touch is essential for connection to myself and relaxed, open, easygoing connections with others.

8. **Ask Questions.** It's important to feel connected, not only to myself but to people around me, people I care about and admire. So ask people how they are doing. Take an interest in their lives. I will often make myself available to others. It's good for me, too; it helps me feel inspired, grounded, connected, and useful.

9. **Check In.** I strive to be honest with myself about my progress. Since I am recovering from a control issue—an eating issue or disorder—I will check in with myself every few months to see how things are going. I will talk with my close friends about how I feel in my skin and give myself the time and space to check in.

10. **Define. Test. Refine. Repeat.** My rules aren't final. I will live by the advice of my good friend and mentor Jeremy Moon: Define. Test. Refine. Repeat. This is one of my favorite pieces of advice. I will check back in with my rules in a few months, and if they aren't the rules for me then, I will define, test, refine, and repeat.

So there you have it. Those are my rules. And now I'll give you the one and only rule you have to follow: make your own rules. It works. With this one rule as a starting place, I maintain a strong, radiant, healthy body from the inside out. I enjoy a clear, focused, engaged mind. I am excited and interested in life and my role in it. I am open to change and appreciate the uniqueness of connecting with the people I meet and expanding my contribution to the world. I'm not afraid to be me, and I'm not afraid to make my own rules.

JUST A SUGGESTION: THROW AWAY YOUR SCALE

Several years ago when I was on my path to getting healthy, I realized I still had a big problem. I was weighing myself several times a day purely out of habit. Weighing yourself, I've found, is a sickness—it's a completely unnecessary routine and a destructive habit. If you have a serious health problem or need to monitor your weight for some valid reason, please listen to your doctor and ignore my advice here. For the rest of you, trust me, you don't need that evil box sitting in your bathroom. Walk on over there and throw it in the trash. Promise yourself that you'll never buy another one. Take the trash out, and that's that. Go ahead. I'll wait.

Did you do it? I hope so! Welcome to the Make Your Own Rules Revolution, where you'll be intuitive, strong, capable, and radiant from the inside out. This isn't just about feeling good on the inside. You'll also look fantastic on the outside. You're on your way, and I'm excited for you!

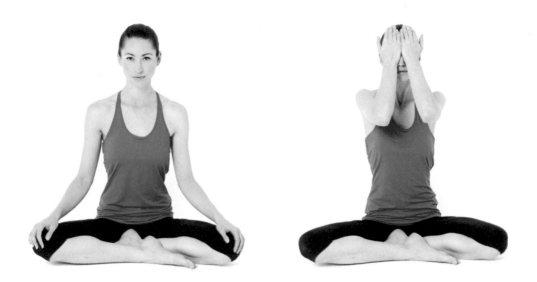

GOAL SETTING

Before you can go about setting your own rules, you have to know what you're aiming for. It's time to set some amazing goals to reach and blow past. I've got a nice, calming practice for you to sensitize to how you feel right now, to make goal setting effortless and authentic to what it is you truly desire. I'm excited for your feeling transformation!

Close your eyes and start to bring your attention to your breath. Notice your inhales and exhales as they come and go. Notice the soft space in between your breaths. Pay attention to how your body feels. Pay attention to how your mind feels. Pay attention to how you feel.

Rub your palms together quickly to create some heat. Once you have some heat, gently press the heels of your hands onto your eyelids and rest your fingers on your forehead. Take three big deep breaths. When you are ready, relax your hands down on your thighs.

Keeping your eyes closed, pay attention to how you feel right now. However you feel—calm, agitated, comfortable, or squirmy—simply take notice. If there is a particular area that feels tense, bring your attention to that area with your mind, take a few big deep breaths, and focus on relaxing that area. If there is another area that feels tense, repeat the deep breaths, and focus on relaxing that area. Hang here for ten long, deep breaths. When you are ready, gently open your eyes.

Time to get down to the business of goal setting. Let's focus on how you feel now and how you would like to feel. Feel free to break out your journal or a notepad and get your thoughts and feelings on paper so you can stay inspired to keep on your great path. If you aren't the journaling type, no need to force it, just ask yourself the following questions and let your answers and feelings soak in.

Remember, it's important to get honest here. I'm not auditing you, so please don't feel judged. This work is for your eyes only. You start where you are, so knowing what's going on with you right now is essential.

Rise and Shine: It's 7 A.M. How do you feel? Do you wake up feeling refreshed and excited for the day? Do you wake up feeling sleepy and groggy and dreading the day? Are you somewhere in between? Does your mood and energy level vary day to day? How do you feel and is it different from how you would like to feel?

Good Midmorning: It's 10 A.M. How do you feel? Are you energized, sluggish, or usually still asleep? What do you typically consume in the morning? Are you all about your morning coffee and bagel or more of a green juice, protein smoothie regular? Do you run on an empty stomach? How do you feel and is it different from how you would like to feel?

Lunchtime: It's noon. Where are you, what are you doing, and how do you feel? What are you having for lunch? How hungry are you around lunchtime? Do you feel tired or alert? Are you moody, cranky, or a ball of sunshine? How do you feel and is it different from how you would like to feel?

Midafternoon: It's 3:30 P.M. What's going on? How are you doing? Are you hanging in there? Are you at work, home, or out? Are you on an adventure? Have you taken any time for yourself yet today? Gotten your yoga and meditation in? Are you reaching for a coffee, cookie, or big glass of water? How do you feel and is it different from how you would like to feel?

Early Evening: It's 7 P.M. What's for dinner? Are you staying in and cooking, going out, or picking up something on the way home? What's the plan for the evening? Are you working late, hitting up a yoga class, having date night, surfing the web, watching TV, or taking a long bath? How do you feel and is it different from how you would like to feel?

Nighttime: It's 10 P.M. What are you up to? Are you cuddled up in bed with a book, working late, checking e-mail, or something else? Are you hungry, stuffed, satisfied, scrounging for a snack? How do you feel and is it different from how you would like to feel?

Midnight: It's 12 A.M. Are you tucked away and off to dreamland, or still up? If you are up, what are you doing? Working, reading, worrying, eating, or something else? If you are still up, when will you get to sleep? Do you have a hard time falling asleep? Do you stay asleep or wake up during the night? How do you feel and is it different from how you would like to feel?

How did that exercise go? Did you learn anything about yourself? Are you happy with your lifestyle and habits, or is there room to feel better? If you found specific things that you'd like to change, keep these in mind when you're making your new rules. If you found things that were good, make sure to keep those when you make your new rules. Now let's jump in and make some rules!

THE KICK START PRACTICE GUIDE

Making your own rules is an empowering practice. When you get comfortable tuning in, following your intuition, and letting it guide you to your own unique path of radiant happiness, there is no turning back. It sounds simple enough to make your own rules, but there is an efficient and fun process of tuning in that will help you know exactly what the best rules are for you right now. The more you practice tuning in, the easier it gets, and soon you'll know exactly when it's time to break another rule and start fresh. Get ready to transform your life!

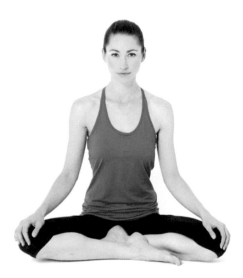

STEP 1: GET CONNECTED. Sit and meditate. Simple meditation is a practice that will sensitize you to how you feel. When you are in feeling mode instead of thinking mode, you are connected to your intuition and in the right place to begin making your own rules. (We'll get into this a lot in the following pages. I want you to get excited about carving out time in your day to check in with yourself.) Your highest purpose is resting right inside you. Tap in, have a listen, and allow your intuition to expand.

TRY IT NOW! Wherever you are, take a moment and get comfortable. Sit up tall through your spine. Close your eyes and rest your hands on your thighs. Allow your body to sway gently side to side and round and round with the aim of finding a neutral, balanced place. Begin to notice your breath as it naturally comes and goes, inhaling and exhaling through the nose. Start to lengthen your inhales and deepen your exhales. Allow your attention to drift inward. If you start thinking or wandering away from your breath, gently guide your attention back to it. If you start to wander again, guide your attention right back again. Don't worry about being perfect or having no thoughts or a clear mind. Simply focus on watching your breath and guiding your attention back when it strays. The process of guiding your attention has movement, is fluid, and changes moment to moment. Continue breathing for a few moments, and, when you're ready, gently open your eyes.

Step 2: Shed What's Not Serving You. Make a list. In your journal, on a scrap of paper, whatever is handy, pick up a pen, marker, or crayon, and write it down. What are the actions that you do and the rules that you follow that aren't serving you? It can be as simple as eating too much sugar or participating in a toxic relationship. These are the things you discovered when you were setting goals in the last section. It's important to face what's not serving you before you can write any new rules.

TRY IT NOW! Grab something to write on and something to write with and start jotting. Be honest with yourself. This list is for you, not to present at an interview. You start where you are, and that's a great place to be. If you're not honest about where you are, you'll be starting where you aren't, and it's hard to get anything done from a place where you aren't. Once you get all of those old behaviors out of your system and onto the paper, they are one step closer to being out of your life for good. Congratulations—today you'll begin to untangle the sticky web of someone else's rules and create a whole new uncharted path of your own. You're about to go where no one has gone before.

step 3: Make Space. Without space, there is no room for inspiration, creativity, or anything new. Declutter your living space. Clean up your social and work calendar.

TRY IT NOW! Why wait till guests come over to make things nice at home? You're worth impressing, too! If you have a home computer, take ten minutes to brush up and organize files into folders and organize the items on your desktop. Doesn't that feel better? Feels more spacious, right? Do the same with your living room, bedroom, and other areas of your home that could use some attention. Don't worry about deep cleaning and clearing out the closets for now, just organize and put things in their places. Fluff pillows and make your home nice for yourself. It really makes a difference. Our surroundings influence our mood and how we feel about things, so if it is in your power to create an inspiring setting to live in, go for it!

step 4: Allow Creativity. Find something you like that is creative and fun. It can be anything: knitting, cooking, yoga, or hiking. We'll be doing a lot of yoga together soon, so if your life is pretty full, don't feel pressured to pick up and enjoy a new hobby, unless of course you feel the inspiration. Let it be an activity that fuels you mentally, physically, emotionally, and spiritually.

TRY IT NOW! You don't have to plan the world's biggest DIY craft project or cover your living room in glitter (unless you really want to—don't let me hold you back). Allow your mind to wander and dream about something to do that is simple that will create space for creativity. Maybe it's doodling, painting, dancing, or writing. It can be anything. A few years back I was walking in Soho on a writing break, looking for some creativity and fresh air. I discovered a shop window filled with candy-colored, fuzzy, thick alpaca wool and superfun hats and sweaters. Inside the shop it was like Christmas; smiling, happy people were knitting magical creations around a table. It was fun, fresh, and cool. This wasn't your grandmother's knitting store, but it had the comfort of Grandma's home. I was so drawn in by the feeling of cozy meets inspiration. The colors, the creativity, the tangibility, it was all so satisfying. I wanted to add that to my life immediately! I got myself a starter kit, watched some online videos, and started creating at home. I knit on the road, too, and it gives me a great sense of calm and ease and inspiration. New ideas pop up during the process, and, row after row, the stress melts right out of my system. The repetition is a lot like meditation and yoga. Maybe you'd like to give knitting a whirl if you're not already on the bandwagon. It's fun and fresh and hip and however you make it. Just like anything else.

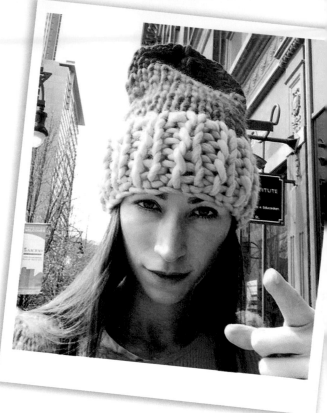

STEP 5: MAKE NEW RULES. Only do this step when you feel ready. You've cleared some space in your life. You've opened up to creativity. You've found what's not serving you. Now you have a solid base from which to formulate your new rules that do serve you and your highest purpose. These can be as simple as planning to prepare your own meals three days a week, or signing up for that yoga membership you keep putting off, or taking steps toward the career of your dreams.

TRY IT NOW! Allow your mind to wander toward what your rules might be for today or for the next 30 days. Perhaps even both! My rules for today are: practice ease at one class at Strala, meditate for at least ten minutes, and set some time for reading and daydreaming. Your turn!

Good job! You've just taken the first step toward creating a healthy and happy you. And remember, one of the great things about setting your own rules is that you can change and evolve them anytime you want. The rules you set for yourself today probably aren't going to be the same rules that work for you next year—they might not even be the same rules that work for you next week or tomorrow.

You'll be able to continually assess what needs to change—what will help you get to where you want to be. And now it's time to take a closer look at the tools that help you stay sensitized so you can update your rules as need be. Exciting!

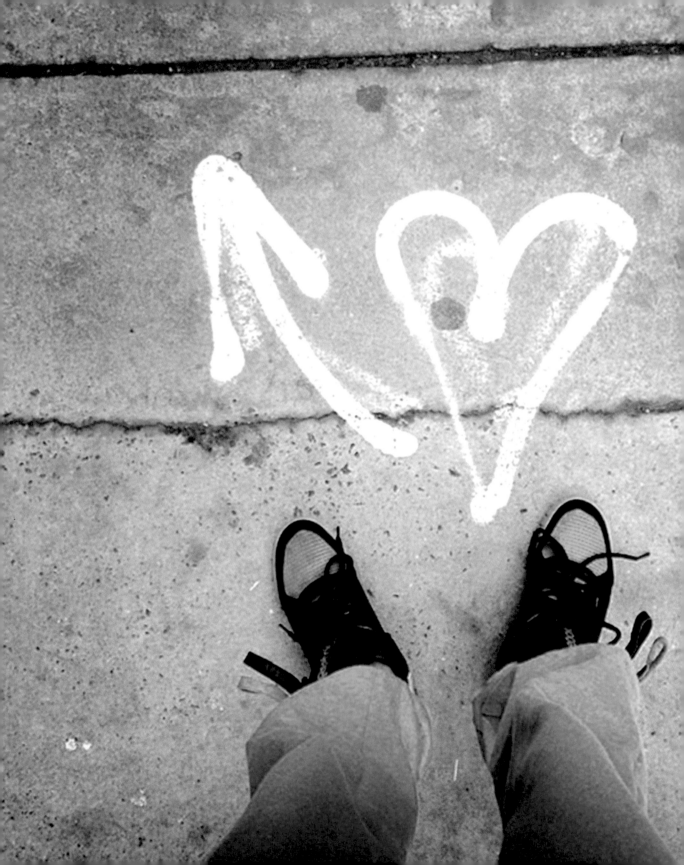

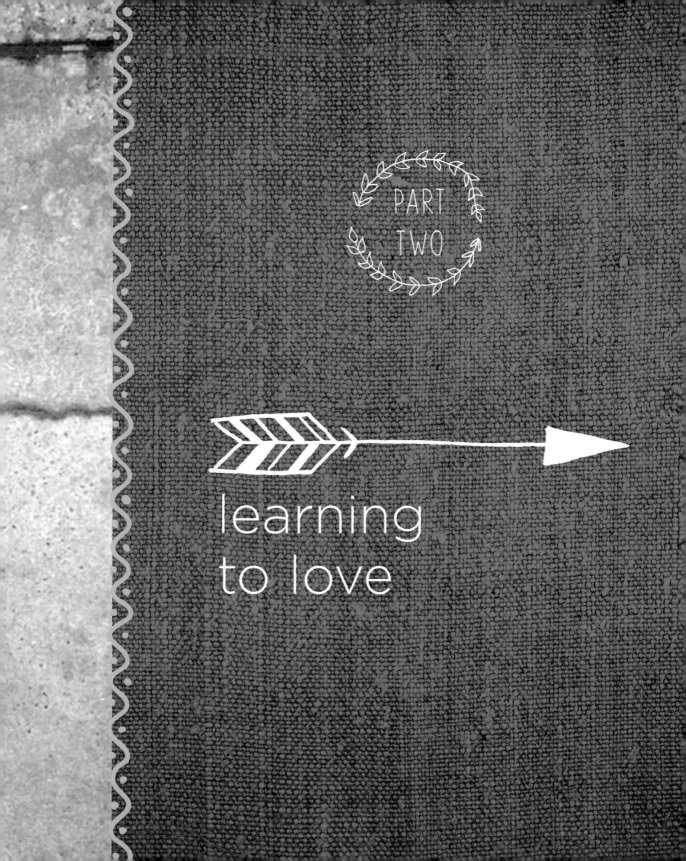

PART
TWO

learning
to love

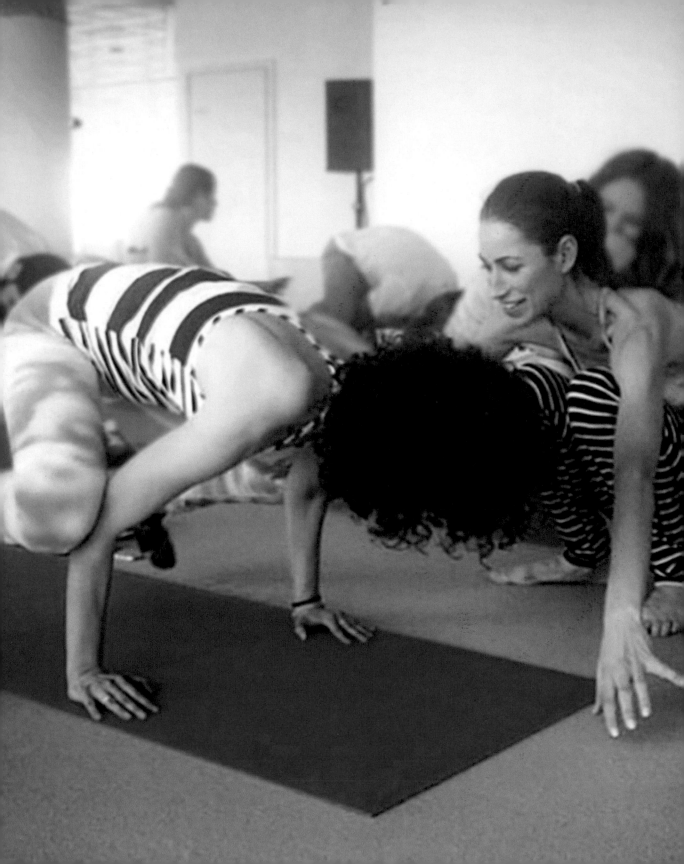

loving your mat

YOU don't have to be flexible. YOU don't have to be able to put your foot behind your head or even touch your toes. You don't have to be able to do a handstand. You don't have to commit hours every day to silent devotion. You don't have to do anything, except be yourself. If you can breathe, you can practice yoga, and you can gain the benefits of a strong, capable body and a calm, focused mind; plus you can be ridiculously happy.

By now, you've probably heard something about the massive benefits of regular yoga practice. Less stress, improved overall health, weight management, improved blood flow, increased strength and flexibility, more energy, more creativity, and the list goes on and on. Seems like the wonder drug, right? The great thing about the health benefits is that they happen from the inside out. The insula is an area of your

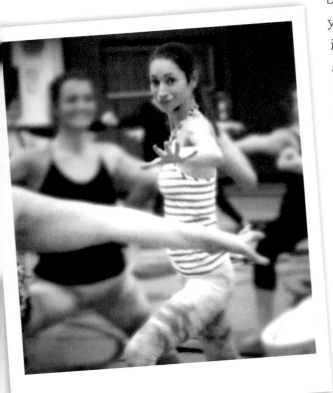

brain located between your eyebrows (what yogis call the third eye). This structure is in charge of your creativity, your intuition, and your overall well-being. Scientists have found that your insula lights up when you practice easygoing yoga and meditation. It strengthens like a muscle, and it tells your body to get healthy. It tells your mind to get creative. It makes you feel happy. It makes you feel like eating veggies over burgers. I'm totally not kidding. You want to lose weight? Don't worry about counting calories; just start practicing easygoing yoga. Your mind will tell your body to crave all the things that are great for you. You will actually *want* to eat spinach. I'm serious! Work your well-being muscle with yoga and become Popeye!

When you focus on an exercise to simply burn as many calories as possible, you turn off your insula and focus on "the burn." Your mind becomes stressed and narrow. Your body becomes tense and stuck. You may burn a bunch of calories by the end of your workout, but you will feel as if you have just survived trauma. Your body and mind go into defense mode to protect you. Problems with digestion and side effects from stress, such as sleep problems and anxiety, prevail. When you go after "the burn," you are also more likely to feel punished and need a reward, which often results in eating a cheat food. It doesn't matter how many calories you burn if you leave your workout and down a burger and a beer. The math just doesn't add up. That said, if you truly enjoy your other nonyoga workouts, you are more likely to gain the benefits of less stress while you perform them. Just make sure you practice something you love—and it's hard not to love yoga when it's all about feeling great from the inside out. This practice is for you!

The physical benefits of yoga almost always come out of a psychological and emotional shift in perspective. How you are in your body is how you are in your life, and yoga is a great tool to check out what's going on with you and then do something positive about it. A young couple from Michigan that came through Strala were so excited to tell me about their transformation from practicing at home daily. Together they had lost more than 400 pounds, which was incredible to hear. Practicing helped them feel great, so they bumped it up to twice daily. They know the real reason for their drastic transformation has to do with how they started to feel. They started to feel incredibly good. They described feeling their bodies buzzing for the first time in a long time. They wanted to treat their bodies well, so they started eating superclean and healthy, filling their diets with fruits and veggies and whole foods. They noticed they didn't want to eat junk anymore because it made them feel dull. They want to keep the great feeling going, so they cook all the time now and have a blast taking care of their bodies and each other. What an inspiration. They had so much energy and vitality when I met them that it was absolutely contagious. We all hugged and jumped for joy.

You can experience a shift like this, too. Just remember, the goal of yoga is to feel great. Don't worry about the poses. Don't worry about the breath. Don't worry about your outfit. Don't worry about anything. Just allow yourself to believe the goal is to feel great. That's it. Simple and awesome. Interested yet?

If you already have a regular yoga practice, then you're all set. Please go out and inspire your friends and family to get on their mats and move with ease every day so they can feel as great as you do. If you have tried yoga, but it hasn't stuck, no worries. I'll help you start where you are, because that's right where you need to be. And I'll help you find what you love rather than what others have told you to do. If you are brand-new to this whole yoga thing, that's exciting, because there is so much you are about to experience and uncover. You are about to cultivate a strong, healthy, and open body from the inside out. You are about to gain a calm, focused, and sharp mind full of creativity. And, maybe best of all, you are about to gain a zest for life and energy to do anything you desire and probably a whole lot more. With regular practice, anything is possible. I'm excited for you.

DON'T BE A POSER

Something funny happens in yoga. Well, actually, let's be honest—a lot of funny things happen in yoga. When you get a bunch of people bending and stretching and acting very serious about it all, there is material for funny. Kidding aside though, often people start practicing yoga because they want to feel better and be less stressed, more connected with themselves, healthier, or stronger. But soon they fall into the trap of desperately wanting to nail a pose. How we see yoga in the world today is in pictures of poses. Although these are a nice way to inspire and invite people into the practice of yoga, pictures of extreme contortionistic shapes can be intimidating and turn people away from practicing because they think they can't do the pose or just plain aren't interested. The other problem they pose (pun intended) is that they sway people to really-really-really want to do that pose. There is nothing terribly wrong with attempting fun yoga poses and even being interested in working up to doing a crazy pose like a handstand, but it's important not to fall into the trap of chasing the poses. They are just poses. The yoga is in feeling your way into you, and the poses are simply something to do.

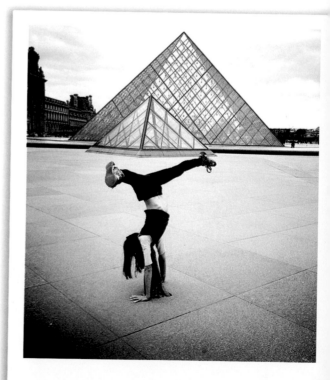

make your own rules diet

Now here's the kicker. It's true that by practicing poses for years, you will probably be able to do some of them. But by practicing feeling into yourself, you'll have achieved something much greater than yoga poses; you'll have found a path into following your intuition and cultivating a strong, radiant, healthy body and a calm, focused mind. And I've got one more surprise for you. Using the feeling approach, you'll be able to do a lot more poses than if you use the posing approach. With the feeling approach, you'll never get injured or feel tense while practicing. With the feeling approach, you'll be able to accomplish hard things easily. Let's start feeling!

HOME PRACTICE

Yoga at home is a wonderful gift you can give to yourself every day. It's your time to check in and get intuitive. One of the many awesome things about practicing yoga at home is that you can do it on your own time, around your own schedule, and for as long (or as briefly!) as you want. Plus you can tailor the kinds of practices you want for your life in each moment. At Strala, we always encourage people to do what feels right in the group setting. But in your living room, you can take feeling to a whole new level. It's all about you! You can even stay in your pj's if you want! I guess pj's are totally acceptable at the studio, too, but you get what I mean. Your practice, your schedule, your dress code, your house! Can't get any more convenient.

The potential missing element you would get from practicing yoga in a class is the support of the group and the guide. Not to worry, I'm right here with you. You have my support every step of the way. You're not getting rid of me that easily. There are six routines laid out in this book, but I also have hundreds more on YouTube (youtube.com/tarastilesyoga) that you can use to keep your practice fresh and interesting. And I'm right there on the other side of the computer ready to answer any questions and chat whenever you wish! So please reach out. I want to hear from you and keep the progress alive and fun. I'm so excited for your journey inward. So many awesome discoveries are waiting for you to uncover them. I'm excited for all the priceless jewels and cool things you're about to find right inside you!

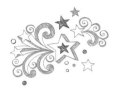

THREE TIPS
TO CULTIVATING
A REGULAR HOME PRACTICE

Now that I hopefully got you all jazzed up, it's time to make a plan so you can ensure feeling connected and inspired is a regular thing instead of a nice idea.

TIP 1

Make space. One of the many awesome things about yoga is how simple it is. Not just the "if you can breathe, you can do it" part, but also the simplicity of what tools you actually need to practice. All you need is you. You don't need any equipment. If you have a yoga mat, great, but you can also practice on the floor—hardwood, tile, carpet, whatever. And the only space you need is how much it takes for you to lie down flat. You can literally practice anywhere. However small your living space is, you have enough room. The foot of your bed is enough! It's good to know you are enough, and you have enough to begin. That's deep, right? Take a look around your home and find your spot. Maybe it's a nice nook in your living room or den, or maybe it's the space beside your bed. Claim your yoga spot, and you're on your way. If you decide to use a yoga mat, roll it out and keep it in your spot. If you're okay with having it out all the time, it's a great reminder. If you walk by your yoga mat and it's rolled out waiting for you, you are more likely to practice. If it's jammed in the back of your closet behind all your winter coats and old sweaters, you're likely to leave it there. If you don't want to keep your mat out full-time, roll it up and keep it near where you practice. Rest it against a wall or a bookshelf. Find a nice spot out in the open where you'll see it and be reminded to take some deep breaths and of the greatness that is inside you.

TIP 2

Schedule it. When you have a date to meet a friend for lunch, or a scheduled work meeting, an interview, or a doctor's appointment, it's in your calendar. Self-care and yoga practice can be the last things to actually go in your schedule as firm appointments, and these are often the first things to get brushed off when your schedule gets full. We are aware of the problem, so fix it. Get your practice in your schedule. Treat your yoga practice just like you would treat any appointment. And don't look at it as taking time out of your life. In fact, it's just the opposite in the long run. You'll be able to prevent health issues, so you won't need as many doctor's appointments. You'll be more creative and inspiring and have more energy to catch up with your bestie on that lunch date, and you will be experiencing rejuvenated blood flow to your brain and be extra sharp and focused in your meetings and interviews. Knowing all the benefits of your practice, how can you brush it off? Get it in your calendar and, trust me, you can find the time. Five minutes today in the morning, ten minutes when you get home from the office or when the baby is napping. Keep it regular, and you'll feel like a superhero in no time. The more you practice, the better you feel, so get your practice in your schedule ASAP. Enjoy!

TIP 3

Do what you can. I'll keep reminding you of this forever: don't worry about being in the perfect picture of a pose. The goal is to feel, not to pose. It's easy to get wrapped up, once you get moving, in wanting to be "good at yoga." The reality is that being good at yoga has everything to do with what's going on inside you—how you are feeling, how your mind is, how at ease you are in yourself—and very little to do with what your posing looks like. Yes, it's important to be safe and not to harm yourself when you practice, but when you practice moving with ease, you'll never force your body into something it's not ready to do. Go after feeling and ease, and the movements will be simple. Soon you'll see the truth in what I'm saying: It's not about the poses. The real yoga is happening on the inside.

HOME PRACTICE CHECKLIST

☐ **Space.** Identify your yoga space. Claim it for your practice. Clear the area of clutter, and place your mat down (if you are using a mat). You might want to keep a notebook handy to write down any great ideas that come to you during your inspirational practices.

☐ **Routines.** If you have been doing yoga for a while, you might feel comfortable making up your own routines. If so, have a blast! If you would like to move along with me, I'm happy to take you for a ride. Starting on page 79, you can find some routines to get you started on your yoga adventure, and you can always find me on YouTube for countless more routines. I promise to keep you on an adventure with yourself for a long time.

☐ **Music.** Music is a personal choice. All the classes I lead, unless it's by the ocean, which is amazing natural music, have really fun music. I find it helps everyone relax, move with the breath, and have a good time. If you love music, feel free to pop in your favorite playlist and have a great time flowing to the beat. You make the rules.

☐ **You.** All you need to get started is you. It's going to be great. You're going on an adventure, and only great things will happen. You're going to have so many insights. You'll gain a superstrong body and an easy, focused mind; plus you'll be building all the tools to get connected and plugged in anytime.

YOU GET WHAT YOU PRACTICE—
CONFESSIONS FROM THE GYM

I want to stress once again that practicing with ease is essential for success. I experienced this in my own life when I got talked into working with a personal trainer. When I was 21, I modeled in an advertisement for a gym chain, and I got a membership out of it. It was a sweet deal for me. I used it to frequent yoga classes and hang in the steam room. If you've ever spent a lot of time at a gym, you might be familiar with the personal trainers roaming around coaxing members into signing up for sessions. One of the trainers always teased me about my yoga thing and challenged me to work out with him, thinking I couldn't keep up. Of course, always up for a challenge and usually a little feisty, I accepted. (Just for the record, there are tons of amazing personal trainers out there—many are good friends of mine—so please know that this is not an anti–personal trainer rant.)

During my first session, I was instructed to push hard, lift weights until I couldn't anymore, and wince and groan when it got tough. I went along for the ride, enjoyed moving my body in different ways, and found it all pretty entertaining at first. I pushed and I lifted and I squatted until my trainer was satisfied. The funny thing was that I didn't get stronger; I only got more disconnected from myself. I felt unsatisfied, tense, and agitated. I felt hungry for foods that weren't healthy or satisfying. I began to eat mindlessly. I began to treat people with less kindness and more carelessness. I felt and acted aggressive because I practiced aggression. After several sessions of humoring my trainer friend, we mutually realized that forcing and pushing weren't for me. We high-fived it out and parted ways. I went back to working on hard things easily and accomplishing hard things easily. My body got stronger and stronger and my eating and treating-people habits returned and became more mindful and kind according to how often I practiced.

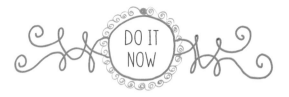

WARRIOR 2 (CALM WARRIOR)

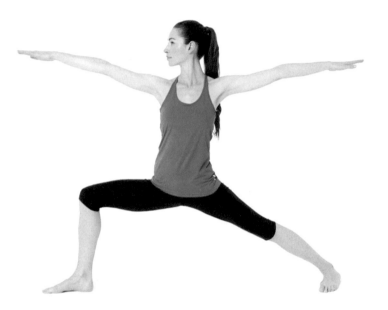

Holding warrior 2 is an interesting practice of calling on your body to work for you just a bit and finding all the places you can relax. It's a great opportunity to ask your mind to be calm and easy under a controlled, expected challenge. When you are calm and easy, you begin to notice how you feel. You have the opportunity to believe in what you feel and the ability to respond to what you feel.

If you can hold warrior 2 for one minute with ease, you can stay calm during other challenging circumstances in your life. That's why it's called practice, not performance. Practicing how you want to be in the movements is more important than the movements themselves. So let's try it.

Step your feet wide apart. Turn your right toes forward and your left toes slightly in toward your body. Bend your front knee until it's over your front ankle. Make sure your knee isn't rolling to one side. It's important to protect your knees. Open your arms to the sides at shoulder height. Look over your right hand. Relax your shoulders. Relax your eyes. Relax your face. Relax your body. Use only the effort you need to stay here. Bring your attention to your breath. Allow your inhales to be long and deep and your exhales a little longer and fuller. Stay here for ten long, deep breaths.

Now let everything relax. Drop your arms down by your sides. Roll around your hips. Let everything be all loosey-goosey. Any tension you are holding on to, whether physical, mental, or emotional, let it drop out and relax. Now, easily, open back into your warrior 2. Hold for another ten long, deep breaths. Change directions and do the same on your other side.

How did that feel? Take note of how your body felt, how your mind felt, and what emotions came up. Was it easier to hold the warrior 2 after rolling around loosey-goosey for a bit? Did you find your body tensing after a while? Were you able to relax and stay movable when tension crept in?

The lesson is that tension is a part of life. We need it in our bodies to a certain degree to be strong, to be able to walk around and accomplish tasks. If we were loosey-goosey all the time, we wouldn't be able to get out of bed. The tension that comes along with anxiety and stress is the part that we can begin to observe and let roll off. We can choose to work efficiently and find more ease in our actions. When we find ease in our actions, our life expands and radiates accordingly.

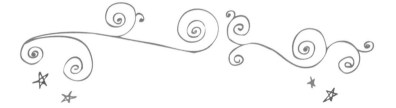

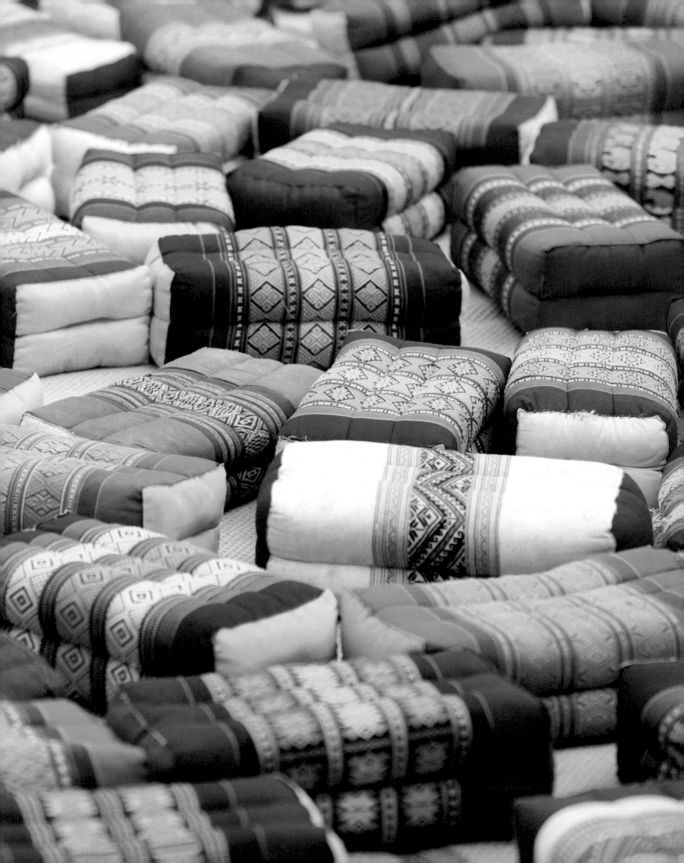

loving
your cushion

Like those of yoga, the benefits of meditation, such as stress reduction, increased sensitivity, and overall health, are becoming more and more recognized—and backed up with research. This makes convincing people to get on the cushion much more fun. Studies have shown what meditators have known for ages: the secret to long-lasting health is in all of this deep breathing and mind calming. Genes that protect from pain, infertility, high blood pressure, and other diseases activate in longtime meditators. Immunity goes up and blood pressure regulates. Many of these benefits have to do with reversing the negative effects stress has on the body. The stress hormones adrenaline and cortisol, which raise the heart rate and weaken immunity, dissolve, making room for happy chemicals, such as serotonin, to flow. In turn, this lowers the heart rate, boosts immunity, and allows the body to radiate. And the benefits increase the more you practice. Good news, right?

Stressful periods of life can be handled effectively with a regular meditation practice. Betty, a regular at Strala, had struggled with eating disorders and clinical depression that had taken over her life for years. Learning how to meditate gave her the tools to slow down and listen, which gave her a chance to hear the negative voices that were rolling around in her head. And with this awareness, she could make a choice to let those thoughts go and put loving, kinder thoughts in. Choosing to remember that we are whole, perfect, and on the right path helps us live in a way that makes life better. Our external worlds get easier and smoother when we pay attention and nurture our internal worlds.

Growing up, I would naturally do what I now know is meditation. I had a lot of room around me, which allowed me to feel an expansive sense of space and calm inside. I found inspiration and creativity in nature. The wonder and magic I found in the nooks and crannies of the forest allowed me to find that same wonder within myself. It was as if I were remembering this practice from somewhere deep inside me. The beauty and calm that surrounded me allowed me to go inside and explore.

Being surrounded by nature is a great place to begin meditation. It makes it easy to be calm, quiet, and connected. We relax easily as the water rolls, the breeze blows, and the clouds drift by. There is always movement that lives inside balance, and nature reminds us that we are okay as the circumstances of our lives change, grow, and expand. The trees bend with the breeze while remaining strong and sturdy. I am nature. You are nature. We have all the same beauty, movement, calm, and peace right inside, waiting to be tapped into.

The honest truth is that we often forget that we are nature. We end up thinking and believing that calm and peace and beauty exist outside us and inside is just the opposite. Inside we become insecure, frustrated, cramped, worried, and stressed. Life is jam-packed, filled with highs and lows, and often has very little or no space to just be. Personally speaking, my life, both work and personal, which to me are the same, is all about creating space. I often get caught with an overflowing plate and have to use what I know and remember. I take a few big deep breaths and make some more space. The space is always there; you just have to tap in and remember. Step off the hamster wheel and find an easier way.

Cultivating a daily meditation practice sets up the foundation that allows you to fall off balance and then roll right back on.

If we are lucky enough to take vacations to relaxing beaches or similar getaways, we remember that sense of calm, ease, and peace from nature. But when vacation is over, we go back to our daily lives and get weighed down again by life's pressures. Schedules, deadlines, goals, workloads, families, oh my!

I know you know what I'm talking about. We are all so busy, and that's just how life is. We decide to fill our time with things we value, and often our leftover time gets filled with other things. Our exterior surroundings might not be an expansive peaceful woods; they might be a busy office, full house, or packed city streets. But the amazing thing about meditation is that when you remember how to tap in, the peace and calm of nature are right there inside waiting, no matter how chaotic your external surroundings might be.

FEELING INTO YOU

What happens when you begin to meditate is that you begin to feel into yourself. You become aware of how you feel physically and emotionally. You start to gain insight into your life and your purpose. Intuition becomes more and more clear, and when you consider your intention, you become a superfeeler.

Meditation practices focus on the breath. There are so many techniques that involve different things to do with the breath. You can count the breath as it comes and goes, holding the breath at the top and at the bottom; breathe short and fast, long and deep, and vary pace and timing to an infinite number of possibilities. The idea behind all the breath work is to allow you to become more aware of yourself in the present moment. When you take a big deep breath, you can feel more than when your breathing is shallow.

Try it now. Wherever you are, close your eyes and take a giant deep breath in through your nose. Hold it at the top for a few moments; then slowly release all the air out through your mouth. Repeat twice more and gently open your eyes.

Imagine if you did more feeling in your daily life and allowed yourself the opportunity to feel your way through circumstances when you weren't meditating. Imagine if you had space between you and whatever is going on in your life. Imagine feeling fully present in the moment, so you could make better decisions. With meditation, you become a sensitized superhero, completely in control, with endless possibilities at your fingertips. When we aren't feeling and aren't meditating regularly, we are subject to our insecurities, mood swings, and negative thoughts. Who can see clearly under all that junk?

Cultivating a daily meditation practice removes the stuff that fogs up your access to your best self. It's like sitting behind a dirty, smeared-up window and one day remembering you can pick up a rag, wipe the window clean, and discover gorgeous scenery on the other side. Better yet, you find out that the window is actually a sliding door and you decide to open the door and take a walk outside. The choice is yours. You can sit in a chair and look at a fogged-up window or wipe away the fog and go exploring.

SPACE TO MEDITATE

Setting up a home meditation practice is even simpler than setting up your yoga practice space. In fact, it can be the same space you use for yoga, which is simply a moving meditation. You might find that you like to practice meditation before or after your yoga practice, so being in the same spot is convenient.

You don't need anything that you don't already have. You can meditate on your couch, sitting up in bed, or even at your desk. However, having a special spot will probably help with familiarity and regularity of your practice. I have two Mexican blankets folded up and placed on the floor against a wall. It's simple, easy, and comfortable, and when I walk by every morning, I see the blankets and remember that if I choose to take five minutes to sit and feel into my breath, my day will be better.

THREE TIPS TO BEGIN
YOUR MEDITATION PRACTICE

Don't worry about clearing your mind. It's easy to fall into the belief that the goal of meditation is to have a crystal clear mind so you can see all the secrets of the universe.

Don't worry; plenty of cool experiences are going to happen to you. There is no need to get wrapped up in getting to everything right away. The mind wanders; that's just what it does. Every time your thoughts carry you off on a journey, just bring your attention back to your breath, back to feeling. That's the practice.

The goal is to notice when your mind wanders. When you notice, you have a choice. You can go along for the ride, or you can guide your attention right back inward. You will do this over and over again. Just see things as they happen. Guide your attention back to breathing and feeling. That's your practice. Make the goal the process, not the destination.

Write it down. If you're anything like me, when you have a lightbulb moment, you don't want to forget it. Exciting thoughts and spontaneous ideas will come to you during meditation. They may be great plans about your business, a creative combination to try out in the kitchen, or your next home project. When these brilliant nuggets pop into your mind, you can either keep diving down the idea train or try to store the ideas in your brain and get frustrated that you had a great idea while you should be meditating. This happened to me time after time, and I finally found a solution. Keep a notebook handy for all those mid-meditation, mind-blowing moments. When a genius idea pops into your mind mid-meditation, take a moment and write it down. Now it's down on paper, and you can come back to it and master plan later. For the next few moments, come right back to your breath. Your lightbulb ideas are now preserved, and your sacred meditation time is intact. Win-win!

Keep it regular. Just like yoga, we can talk about the benefits and understand how great life will be with all this practice, but it only works if you actually do it. And the same rules go here: five minutes is better than nothing, and five minutes a day, every day, adds up to a whole lot. Try it out for one week and you'll feel a big difference. First thing in the morning is a great time to set the habit. You don't even have to leave your bed for this one. Simply sit up, get comfortable, and pay attention to your breath for five minutes. If your thoughts start to take you away from your breath, see if you can guide your attention right back. If your thoughts start to drift again, guide yourself back again. After your five minutes, go about your day as usual and notice if you feel any different. Warning: you might start to see yourself differently, with more compassion; you might start to see others differently, with more compassion; and you might start to see more possibilities in your life. You might even have the desire to help others who could use your support. Get ready for some great stuff to transform you from the inside out.

TO INTEND OR NOT TO INTEND...
THAT IS THE QUESTION

Every time you meditate you have an intention—a reason you are choosing to meditate. And just like breathing variations, there are infinite intentions. Your intention may be to deal with stress by practicing daily meditation, or to help yourself be more compassionate by practicing daily meditation. Considered or subconscious, intentions drive our actions. They work best when they are considered, clear, and simple—just like an order at a restaurant. To order, you would review the menu and then ask for pasta with a side of spinach. Not many people simply walk in and say, "Oh, I don't know. Just give me dinner." You get what you ask for; so make sure you think about what you want and clearly intend to get it. You don't need to pretend to be more spiritual than you are and come up with something fancy like, "My intention is to heal the world." Although that sure is nice, and, who knows, you just might do the trick! You can create an intention as simple as, "My intention is to be more patient toward my little sister when she asks me strange questions." Our actions define who we are, and setting an intention will help us act in ways that we would like to act, so we have the impact we want on our own lives and the lives of others.

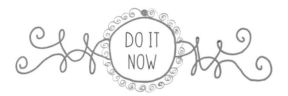

ONE-MINUTE MEDITATION

Sit up straight with a tall back. Make sure you are comfortable. If you are in a chair, place your feet on the ground evenly. If you are sitting on the floor, try crossing your legs or sitting on your heels. Rest your palms in your lap. Close your eyes and begin to pay attention to your breath. Watch your inhales and exhales as they come and go. Allow yourself to become interested in the depth and pace of your breathing. Begin to lengthen your inhales and exhales. If it feels comfortable, pause at the top of your inhale and at the bottom of your exhale.

Allow your face, neck, shoulders, and back to be easy. Allow your hips, legs, and feet to be easy. If you notice your thoughts starting to drift, guide your attention back to your breath. If you notice drifting again, guide your attention back to your breath.

Just like a small child needs to hold your hand to stay safe when she crosses the street, your attention will need you to act as a guide to stay on the right path. Continue to breathe here for ten more long, deep breaths. When you are ready, gently open your eyes.

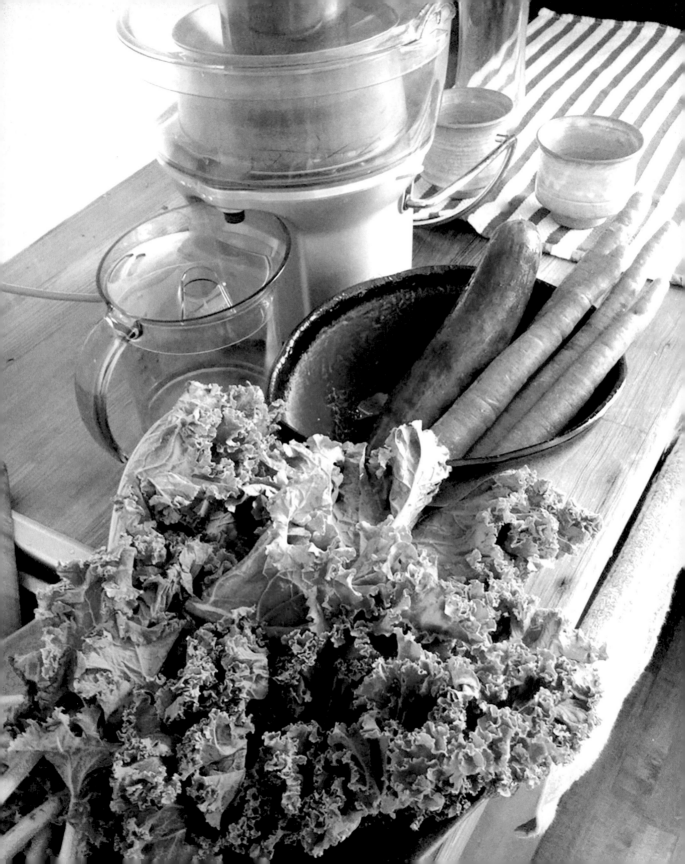

loving
your kitchen

COOKING IS THE SAME AS YOGA AND MEDITATION—IF you can breathe, you can do it! But in this case, perhaps it's more like if you can eat, you can cook. Seriously. It's supersimple. If I can do it, you can do it!

Step one is simply getting yourself in the kitchen, and I don't mean shoveling takeout into your mouth over the sink late at night. When life gets busy, cooking and eating well can be the first thing to go out the window.

As the fridge becomes barren and our schedules packed, takeout and fast food enter the picture and begin their war on our health. It doesn't feel great to consume unhealthy foods, but it happens when we get backed into a corner.

Once you get in the kitchen and get your hands good and dirty, cooking becomes a blast, a creative outlet, and just plain fun. Inventing in the kitchen provides an elevated, lighthearted experience, just like when you were a kid playing around outside, having a good old time rolling around in the mud, climbing trees, and exploring for the sake of adventure. Once you catch the fever of getting messy in the kitchen, cooking starts to become something you schedule time for, just like all of those very important meetings.

Let the goal switch from it being a chore to eat healthy to actually enjoying what you eat and having a great time. Snap on your explorer's hat and get ready for an adventure with the reward of lasting health, energy, and radiance, so you can accomplish your wildest dreams.

Even if you're far off course right now, you can move back to health if you choose to.

FROM GUMMY BEARS TO GREEN JUICE

I grew up eating pretty well, and it was all put right in front of me. My mom kept a nice garden and cooked dinner for our family every night. She packed green peppers and carrots in my lunch instead of processed foods. And she always told me packaged foods were bad for my health, a waste of money, and terrible for the environment. The only good thing was convenience, but it came with a big price.

When I was home and hungry, I would wander into the kitchen to see what Mom was cooking. I'd steal a spoon to grab some cookie dough or try a sauce or a soup before it was ready. Occasionally I would be recruited to wash the dirt off and snap the ends off green beans. On special occasions, such as Thanksgiving, I might be asked (if I was lingering around in the kitchen nibbling) to whip up a bowl of mashed potatoes. I would be closely monitored because I usually made

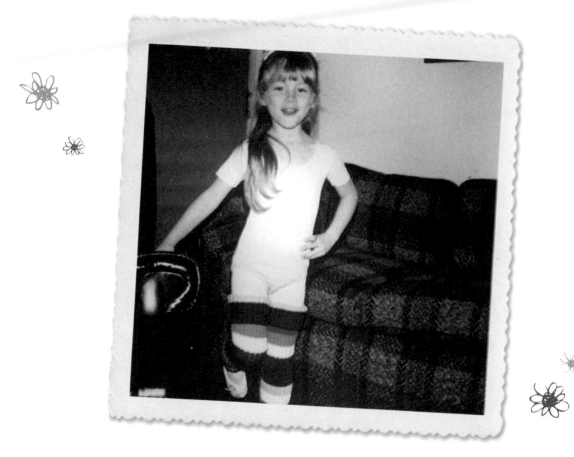

a big mess. Eventually I was demoted to taking drink orders for the extended family. My new, less messy gig was to go around and ask who wanted iced tea, lemonade, water, or milk. (I'm an Arnold Palmer girl myself, always having to make my own rules.) I was stuck in the middle. Not qualified for cooking, not into watching sports on TV. I knew I had a lot to learn in the kitchen but didn't know where to start or what to ask.

During holidays our whole family got together—grandmas, grandpas, aunts, uncles, and all my cousins. We rotated houses, and each holiday was hosted by a different relative. It was a nice system, since almost everyone lived on one long country road. Cooking was the main event, and it was handled by the pros. Mom, grandmas, and all my aunts took care of the main courses, the side dishes, and, oh yeah, the best part, the pies!

Fast-forward out of childhood to young adulthood. After leaving my ballet conservatory in Chicago, I got a one-way ticket to New York City and began to fend

for myself. Even though I had already faced problems with my weight and control issues, being completely in charge didn't lead me immediately to health. In fact, it meant trips to the deli for a Diet Dr Pepper and a bag of mustard-flavored pretzels. A pack of gummy bears or Sour Patch Kids from the newsstand was a suitable on-the-go snack. Fro-yo topped with granola fit into the "totally acceptable dinner" category. A food cart falafel was a complete gourmet meal. Falafel comes with pickles, lettuce, hummus, and hot sauce. That was fancy!

I was spending around $10 a day on meals, satisfying my frugal sensibilities, but all the commonsense, eating-food-that-is-good-for-you philosophy that was instilled in my upbringing went right out the tiny window that directly faced another building in the postage stamp that was my first New York apartment. I knew my creative eating habits and empty cupboard and fridge (minifridge, actually) would eventually catch up with me, but at the time, working and building a life and a career for myself were my first and only priorities. I was having a great time, and taking time to shop for food, prepare meals, and eat well just didn't have a place in my calendar. The thought of taking time to nurture myself seemed like a waste of energy. Taking care of myself fell somewhere in the nonessential to not-very-necessary part of the spectrum.

It's embarrassing to admit, but it must have been a good few years of living in New York before I actually entered a proper grocery store and grabbed a shopping cart. It was a huge step for me, and I was way out of my league.

I nervously navigated my squeaky cart around the aisles, trying to look as though I belonged. I felt like any minute someone would point, laugh, and call me out as an impostor. Surely everyone would drop their groceries and join in the cruel laughter. I was straight-up panicked.

To take my attention away from my horror-movie panic moment, I grabbed a box and started studying. I had no idea what to do with all the green stuff around the edges of the grocery store, so I stayed in the middle, where labels would tell me what to do. Somehow I found the shiny packaging and the clear explanations comforting. The packages told me what would taste great and be healthy for me. All I had to do was purchase, open, occasionally add water, heat up, and eat. I felt safe and formed a new plan: buy foods with directions, follow directions, and eat a little better. Raisin Bran and Progresso soup replaced fro-yo and mustard pretzels. I also discovered cottage cheese and pickles, and this became a special main dish of sorts. Soon I got up the nerve to look at the frozen food section, which meant Tater Tots and frozen pizza. I bought the special ketchup with a spicy kick just to be gourmet. I knew I hadn't figured it out at all, but I knew I was getting closer. At least I wasn't afraid of the grocery store anymore. And just for full disclosure, this grocery-store–anxiety and Tater Tots phase lasted a few years. I'm a quick learner in other areas of my life, but learning all about food and what it means to really be healthy took awhile. Yikes!

I had no idea how unhealthily I was actually eating. I felt sluggish in the mornings, was irritable in the afternoons, and had some trouble sleeping, but I just assumed that's what busy life in the big city was supposed to be like.

It wasn't until I figured out how to revolve my life around helping others with yoga that I started to take care of myself, too.

Once this shift happened, I made sure to steer myself directly onto the path of an interested, curious, experimental adventurer in food and health. I had all sorts of questions, and I wasn't afraid to ask this time. I asked people that I shared yoga with what they ate. I asked people I admired what their favorite recipes were. I started to take a good look at my kitchen. Thankfully at this point I had a full-size fridge to enjoy. I got comfortable along the outside edges of the grocery store (where all the fresh produce is kept). I got friendly with the farmers at the outdoor weekend markets, and I started learning a lot. I got more and more comfortable experimenting and finding ease in the process.

I started creating all kinds of salad variations, making my own dressings, inventing sauces, and blending things. Sometimes it turned out pretty well. Sometimes I let some produce go bad, ate it anyway, and gave myself food poisoning. Not good. It didn't matter to me so much because I wasn't afraid to fail. Failing is better than not trying, and anything is better than a lifelong addiction to Diet Dr Pepper. There was no turning back. I learned a ton of lessons and had a ton of flops in my early green kitchen days, but I know if I had missed any of the exploration, I wouldn't have the freedom and confidence I enjoy in the kitchen today.

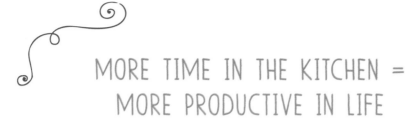

MORE TIME IN THE KITCHEN = MORE PRODUCTIVE IN LIFE

We can talk all about how eating healthier will change our lives. We become clear, focused, sharp, energetic, intuitive, and aware. Our bodies get strong and healthy. We get sick way less often, and we prevent diseases before they have a chance to make a home in our bodies. The studies and books and articles that cover these benefits are endless, and we've all read them. What many don't talk about, however, is that when we schedule time for taking care of ourselves and get into the kitchen, we become much more efficient and productive in the rest of our lives. All that time touching, massaging, chopping, juicing, stirring, and tasting is therapeutic, stress reducing, and creativity promoting. Don't be surprised if you get your next big idea while steaming some spinach or squeezing lemon on some spaghetti squash. This effect may not have been studied by scientists throughout the years, but this is what I've found in my own life and what I've heard from the other folks who have made this switch.

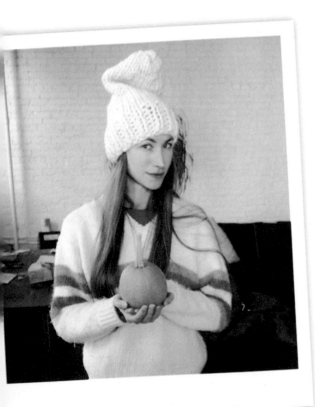

If you are one of the millions who think they are too busy to cook and eat well, just know, once you start and get hooked, you'll have so much more energy and zest to offer everything that is scheduled in your daily planner. You'll have the space in your mind to come up with even more innovative ideas to further your goals. Plus you'll be living in a newly cultivated, radiantly healthy body; have glowing skin; look younger; and be sick of hearing from friends, family, co-workers, and strangers, "Wow, you look great! What's your secret?" Be prepared. It's going to happen and it can happen fast.

 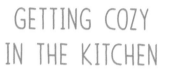 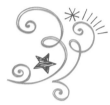

GETTING COZY IN THE KITCHEN

Just like everything else, it's important to start where you are. Being in the kitchen is really fun once you get your hands dirty and let loose a bit. The best part is you are ready to start now. A cooking course is not required, and you don't need to run out to the most fancy and expensive gourmet grocery and buy every gadget on the planet. If you're into kitchen gadgets, that's totally cool, but it's not required to get healthy and happy and have a whole lot of fun. There are two items that I recommend you buy if you can. You'll use these two items over and over, probably every day, and the return on investment will be much greater than your dollars spent. I'm talking about a juicer and a high-powered blender.

In the same vein, many people worry that eating healthy will be too expensive. If you are not interested in going into debt while becoming a healthy, radiant machine, I'm right there with you! Breaking the bank on the path to your most awesome self is completely unnecessary—and unwanted. It would surely cause stress, anxiety, and disease.

The Environmental Working Group (www.ewg.org) has a ton of amazing resources and information about food. My favorite section is "Good Food on a Tight Budget." Even if you're not on a careful budget, it's a great list of the most nutrient-dense foods that come at the lowest costs. Must be my frugal farm, small-town roots sticking with me.

FRIDGE HOVERING

During my canned soup years, not only was I improperly nourishing myself with food, I was also allowing my stress and anxiety levels to soar with no thoughts about needing to change. What I found happening more often than I like to admit was mindless, late-night fridge hovering. Bedtime would roll around, and, instead of hitting the hay, I would start some wacky new project varying from rearranging my closet to going through old photos to watching an indie art film marathon. My projects had goals: find clothes to donate, organize massive stacks of memories, or deepen my art house sophistication. These were justified! However, a few hours into my projects, anxiety would bubble up. I'd wander to the kitchen to see if I had anything to eat. I wasn't really hungry, but I figured that eating something might pacify my anxiety and help me sleep. Unfortunately, many times my fridge hovering led to another can of oversalted canned soup with salty crackers. The more salt, the better.

After my postmidnight snack, I would usually be able to pass out until the morning, only to wake up stuffed, groggy, and not very interested in the day ahead. My eating for the new day was already off to an icky start. Waking up with a full belly is never fun. I would wait out eating until lunch, and by then I would be so hungry that I would end up eating something unhealthy again, maybe a falafel or bowl of cereal. Dinner would be wonky, too, and I'd end up repeating the cycle again and again.

What I learned over the years is that fridge hovering and its consequences can be mitigated in two ways: eating healthy and giving myself proper nighttime care to wind down for a restful sleep.

When I got interested in the kitchen, I started buying fruits and vegetables and making salads, soups, and smoothies. When night rolled around, if I was hungry, I would have some real food that wouldn't leave me feeling gross in the morning. When I woke up, I was hungry for breakfast and would make myself a smoothie or some avocado toast. Eating real food cured me of eating junk all day long.

As for my nighttime routine, I put my phone away, turn the computer off, and sit up in bed for a few minutes and follow my breath. If my body feels cramped from the day, I'll add in a few lying down twists in bed that prepare me for a good rest. It's important to get good sleep because a lot of great things are happening for you while you sleep. Your body repairs itself. Your mind rests and taps into your intuition. You set off to dreamland to create, adventure, and explore. If you don't get good sleep, you probably feel irritable, unsettled, and anxious. Things start to go haywire in your system. When you're sleep deprived, your body isn't able to properly handle the food you eat. Plus you have more cravings for high-calorie, sugar-laden foods—you just need something to get through the day! And then the bad eating habits fuel the bad sleeping habits and the cycle continues. So figure out what works for you. Cozy up with a good book, take a long, hot bath, do some meditation or stretching. Whatever it is, a routine signals your body that it's time for sleep.

FIVE-STEP KITCHEN KICK START

Now that you know that getting your kitchen in shape is totally doable for anyone, here's a nice and easy way to start off on the right foot.

FIVE-STEP KITCHEN KICK START

☐ **Step 1: Take a good look around.** Open the cupboard, fridge, and freezer and take an honest look. What ya got in there? How is your packaged-to-fresh-food ratio? Do you have more cookies, chips, candy, frozen dinners, and ice cream or more fruits, veggies, nuts, and healthy grains?

☐ **Step 2: Toss the junk.** Get your recycle bin and garbage can ready and don't be delicate. Everything must go that isn't good for you. Just get rid of it. We'll start fresh. It might feel wasteful to toss out perfectly good edible calories when people are starving in the world. This is a onetime toss out. It's a fresh start for you and the beginning of your health revolution. You'll become so much more sensitized that you won't be acquiring junk in the future. And don't donate those Ring Dings to the food bank; get yourself healthy so you have more energy to volunteer to deliver healthier options to those less fortunate.

☐ **Step 3: Clean it up.** Now that you've got your recycle and trash bags filled up, it's time to clean everything up and make space for the goodness that is about to enter your life.

☐ **Step 4: Make a list.** Jot down your wish list of fruits and veggies and all your essentials to whip up some wholesome goodness. Make sure you eat a little something before you head to the market to avoid buying a bunch of things you don't need because you're hungry. Trust me—it's easy to grab the cookies and the premade food when you're famished.

☐ **Step 5: Have fun.** Most important, this whole process should be fun. The good part is already happening. You don't have to wait until you throw your first big healthy dinner party. Let yourself have fun with what you're doing now, whether it's clearing out the kitchen of old yucky food products, scrubbing the fridge drawers, or browsing the farmers' market for new and exciting plants to play with. The fun starts now.

STOCKING YOUR KITCHEN

I know that I said I wasn't going to tell you what to eat and how to eat—this is about making your own rules after all. But I also don't want to leave you hanging, so here's a list of some of the things I keep in my kitchen on a regular basis. The foods on this list are included in the Environmental Working Group's website as some of the most nutrient-dense foods for the lowest costs. Eating well can be financially frustrating, but it doesn't have to be when you get resourceful. With just these things, I can easily whip up something healthy and delicious.

DARK GREEN VEGETABLES	
Dark greens are the best. The more you eat and drink them, the more you soak up the pure energy that composes these gorgeous plants. Eat them daily for super energy, glowing skin, and a happy life.	
BROCCOLI	MIXED SALAD GREENS
COLLARDS	SPINACH
KALE	
RED/ORANGE VEGETABLES	
Red and orange veggies are festive and fun. They add tons of vitamins and healing properties to your body and brighten up your plate.	
CARROTS	SWEET POTATOES
PUMPKIN	TOMATOES
GRAINS	
Fill up on these good grains, and you'll be feeling fantastic fast.	
BARLEY	BULGUR
BROWN RICE	OATMEAL

COOKING FATS & OILS

One of the things that makes me feel like a gourmet in the kitchen is having a variety of oils. These are some of my favorites!

CANOLA OIL	SAFFLOWER OIL
EXTRA-VIRGIN OLIVE OIL	SOYBEAN OIL
PEANUT OIL	

BEANS & PROTEINS

I love mixing beans and lentils together in glass jars and preparing them with veggies. You really can't go wrong. Topped with some fresh lemon or soy sauce, these make a fantastic, nutrient-dense, and satisfying meal.

BLACK BEANS	MUNG BEANS
CHICKPEAS	PINTO BEANS
LENTILS	RED KIDNEY BEANS
LIMA BEANS	

NUTS & SEEDS

I carry these nuts mixed together during the day to have as snacks when I'm on the go. Also amazing in any salad and other dishes.

ALMONDS	PECANS
HAZELNUTS	SUNFLOWER SEEDS
PEANUTS	WALNUTS

BASES & SPICES	
Try to buy your spices in small amounts so they don't go stale. Ethnic and farmers' markets carry spices at good prices. The best way to save is to grow your own! I have a fire escape filled with basil. The seeds cost me less than $2 for an unlimited supply!	
CAYENNE PEPPER	PEANUT BUTTER
CINNAMON	PEPPER
DIJON MUSTARD	SALT
GARLIC	SOY SAUCE
HONEY OR BROWN SUGAR	STOCKS FOR SOUPS
LEMON JUICE	VANILLA EXTRACT
LIME JUICE	VINEGAR
ONIONS	WHOLE-WHEAT FLOUR

WHAT I AVOID

If you knew me a few years ago, I would have looked at you sideways if you told me I was going to get rid of the following list from my regular intake, but here we are. I have more energy than I did when I consumed more of this stuff, and I'm a healthier, happier me, so I'm not going back. I'm not an extreme person. I do have these things occasionally; I just recognize they make me feel not so great, so I stay away for the most part and gravitate toward things that make me feel fantastic. Seems like a no-brainer, but the cycle is the thing to break. Thankfully all that "feeling better with easygoing yoga and meditation" works to steer us in the right direction. I also have this really sweet rule: whenever I'm in someone's house whom I care about, and he or she serves me something, I eat it. When food is made with love, it has a whole other set of healing properties you just can't get even in the most perfect organic broccoli stem on the planet. This rule makes going home for the holidays full of love and no arguments. Lectures about converting everyone to eat greens don't need to exist. Families listen more than we may know, and they appreciate when you eat their potato salad and pie. They're filled with love.

Dairy: I keep my dairy consumption to a minimum because I notice a phlegmy voice the morning after I drink or eat it. Plus, I just don't feel as clear as usual. I call it my dairy hangover. Bloating, fuzzy head, and a clogged-up voice isn't the best feeling. Studies have also shown that consuming mass quantities of dairy is not great for overall health. For everyday use, almond milk is in my fridge. It's great in tea and coffee, for baking, and with cookies! Also I'm spoiled in New York. You can get almond or soy milk at any coffee shop and most restaurants. If you really want to be crafty, you can make your own almond milk pretty simply. Homemade almond milk lasts for a few days in the fridge, so make only what you'll want to go through in less than a week.

Meat: I'm not a meat eater anymore. When I started cooking for myself, it was simply easier not to buy and prepare meat. So I didn't. And then over time, eating vegetarian made me feel stronger and more energetic. I just didn't feel like eating animals. I didn't feel it was necessary for me. There are plenty of proteins and nutrients in dark greens, beans, lentils, and nuts to sustain me and create a healthy, radiant body and mind.

   The more you live well, practice yoga and meditation, and eat veggies, the more eating plant-based food simply feels great. You're of course free to make your own decisions on what is best for you and your family. If not eating completely vegetarian, I would recommend limiting your meat intake and making sure that the meat you do ingest is high quality and humanely raised. These meat products generally have less fat and are more filling. They also aren't pumped full of artificial hormones and antibiotics. Plus, these practices are way better for the environment—and the animals.

BOOZe: Don't worry, a heavy sermon isn't coming. I'm not going to turn into a nagging parent, and I'm not going to tell you what to do. This is just my little story.

When I first moved to New York, I thought drinking was what I was supposed to do. Go out, meet people, and pretend like you enjoy it. The key word for me is pretend. Sometimes it's just easier to go with the flow, and alcohol can make you feel more confident. But when I stopped following my intuition about how much to drink, I got a little lost. Thankfully I never developed a serious problem, and, once I shifted my attitude, my desire to drink faded. Some people aren't so lucky. What starts out as having fun leads to reckless behavior that drives a lifelong addiction. Being a boozer isn't classy, isn't pretty, and does nothing good for you—and I don't really need to remind you of all the empty calories contained in booze and mixed drinks.

For me, alcohol is now a treat. I have an occasional glass of wine at a special dinner. It's not an everyday habit necessary to relax. I know that everyone needs to go through their own experiences with drinking, so consider my lecture finished. Just know that you are awesome, just as you are, without the booze.

So there you have it. I hope I've shown you that the kitchen isn't nearly as scary as you might think. Mastering your perfect combinations and meal plans might take some time and experimenting, but it's fun. As long as you don't expect to cook a five-star feast on the first try, you'll be fine. And then, once you can, you'll enjoy it so much more because you'll remember all the little moments that led you there.

It's good to be different, and it's great to be you! With cooking, just aim to cook like you, not someone else. When you start to explore in the kitchen, your cooking style, your comfort level, and your process develop and become uniquely yours—and your creations are uniquely special. Who cares if your pancakes turn out mushy or burned? Who cares if your pasta dish doesn't turn out like the cookbook picture? The more you experiment, the more comfortable you'll be inventing and the more fun you'll have.

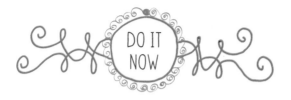

GREEN JUICE

One day in my exploration, a big sign knocked me over the head in the most fun and loveliest of ways. I met Kris Carr, superstar, wonder woman, and plant activist, who was diagnosed with cancer at age 31. She had very publicly documented and transformed her life and her health using food as medicine, inspiring millions along the way—including me.

Kris's transformation was something I desired for my own health, and I was so happy that synchronicity stepped in to give me a boost. We met when we were shooting a YouTube video together, and throughout the shoot I gushed over her and asked her a million questions. She must have known I needed help, and soon after we met, a juicer showed up in the mail. It was a sign—a sign that just showed up at my apartment and came with instructions. There was no more messing around. It was time to take this to the next level and get to juicing the greens. I recorded my first juicing attempt for a YouTube video and was a little afraid the juicer was going to eat me. After a few spins with the juicer, I got more cozy with it and started whipping up all kinds of awesome green combinations and, as a result, enjoyed the straight-up life energy shots with every gulp. Here's what juicing has done for me:

1. **Party on the inside.** My whole internal world got happier when I drank the green love. Dark leafy greens are rich in antioxidants that cleanse your body of stored wastes and toxins that get in the way of proper cell and organ function. It's like a car wash with the works for your insides. Benefits include improved digestion, upped energy levels, easier weight loss and weight management, and overall feeling supergreat.

2. **Get alkalized!** Imagine it's a hot summer day. There is a gorgeous swimming pool right in front of you. You're in your suit and ready to jump in. You leap in without a care. The water is perfect, not too cold,

not too hot. It rushes over you as you swim around. That's how I like to think of an alkalized body. Perfect conditions outside and inside. Things feel awesome and work great. On the flip side, have you ever been in a pool with way too much chlorine and an iffy temperature? That's like having a system filled with too much acidity, which we get from eating fried foods, meats, sugars, caffeine, and salts. One of my favorite things about drinking green juice is that it brings your pH balance back to normal, which means you don't crave the fried foods, meats, sugars, caffeine, and salts that messed you up in the first place. You won't even have to try to resist your favorite junk foods when you start putting the greens in the juicer.

3. **secrets to the universe revealed.** Okay, this may feel a little out there, but when I drink green juice I get the same fuzzy awesome feeling I get when I have a really great yoga practice or a really insightful meditation session. I feel creative, inspired, and connected to myself and my surroundings.

SO NOW THAT YOU KNOW THE BENEFITS, MAKE SOME JUICE!

THE KERMIT

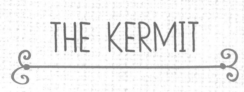

SERVES 2

4 big stalks kale with stems, torn into manageable pieces, or 4 cups spinach
2 stalks celery
1 cucumber
¼-inch fresh ginger, peeled

Juice it up and enjoy!

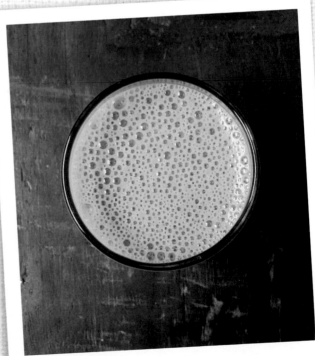

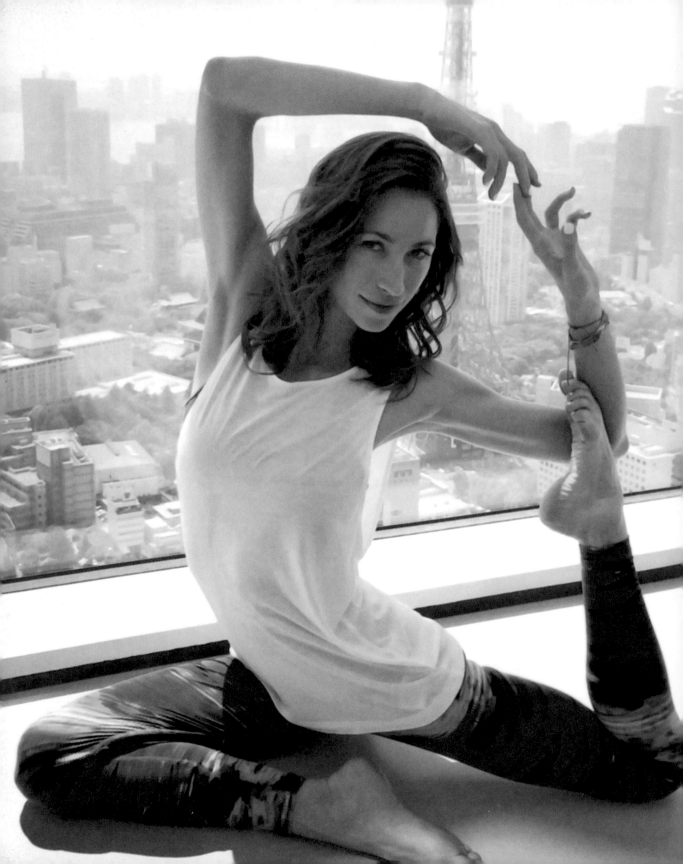

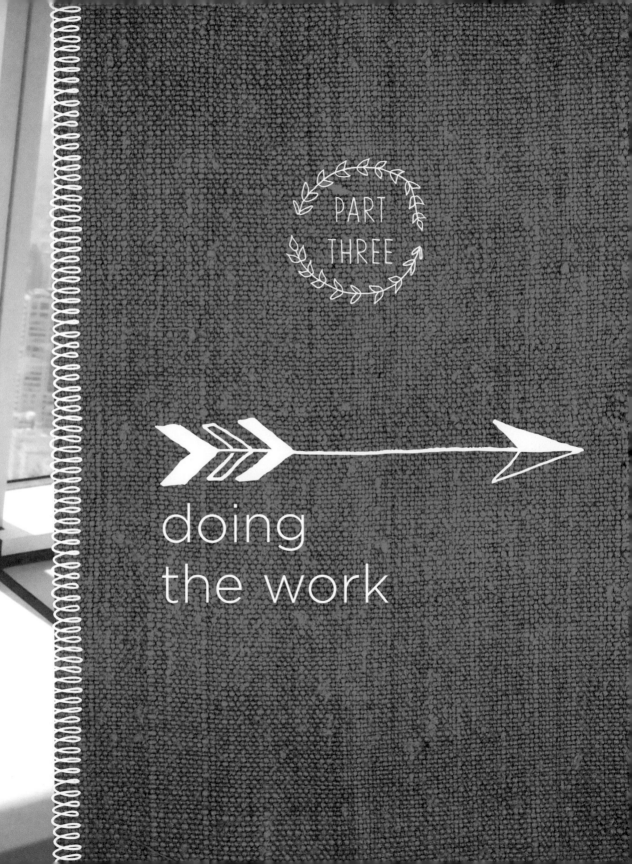

PART
THREE

doing
the work

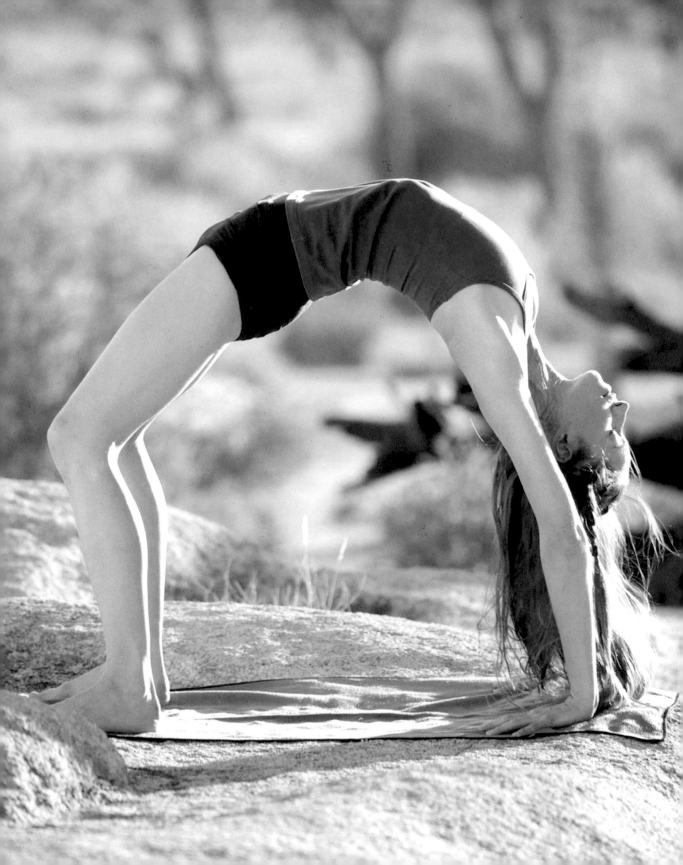

working your mat

One of my favorite things about having a regular yoga practice is knowing that every time I step on my mat I'm going to feel better—no matter what. If I already feel great, I'll feel even better. If I don't feel so good, better is on the way. It works every time. All you have to do is show up and allow yourself to breathe deeply and move with ease. The goal isn't to wrap your foot around your head and balance on one finger; it's simply to feel better. The poses and movements are there to help along the way.

Our experience in life has everything to do with how we feel. How we feel informs what we think, how we treat ourselves and others, what we eat, and what we do with our time. Even the cells in our bodies react to how we feel. The science of epigenetics shows that we can literally change the way our genes express themselves by what we think, how we feel, what we eat, and what we do with our time. So let's start feeling a whole lot better!

When you go through the routines, allow yourself to move in a way that feels good and to linger where it feels nice to linger. There is no need to be strict and rigid with the poses. Go at your own pace, and move gently with your breath. Let your inhales lift you and your exhales soften you. When your body is relaxed and easy, you'll be able to accomplish so much more with a lot less effort, and you'll feel fantastic from the inside out. Some of the best benefits of yoga happen when your relaxation response and intuition are turned on, and this happens when you allow your body to move with ease and your mind can relax and feel free. If you notice your body and mind getting stiff and tense, take a moment to soften your knees, roll around a bit in your body, take a few big deep breaths, and come back to easy.

I designed several routines to guide you right back to yourself, where all the good stuff is. When you feel better, you'll naturally want to take better care of yourself and eat food that is both nourishing and delicious. You'll start to feel strong, capable, confident, and radiant. You'll have a healthy body and a calm, focused mind. So try out the routines and have fun. Yoga is easy when you stop posing and start feeling. Enjoy the ride!

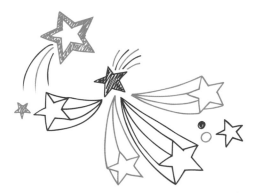

ENERGIZING MORNING FLOW: WAKE UP AND GET MOVING

What's better than waking up fresh in the morning, knowing there is a full day ahead with endless possibilities? Know that you have the power to make your day fantastic! Practicing ease of body and mind will help you operate at your best so you can be in control.

The difference between a good day and a great day can literally depend on what you do in those first five or ten minutes after you wake up. I've found the best thing for me—and many of the people I work with—is to dedicate those minutes to my personal well-being. For me, that means I'm on my mat. When going through a difficult phase of life, this daily practice can be a real lifesaver.

I put together this series of movements for you to open and strengthen your body with ease. In the morning, you may feel a little tighter in your body and a little sleepy in your mind, so this routine moves easily with your breath to gently wake you up. It will energize your spine and open your hamstrings, hips, and shoulders to give you a nice spacious feeling in your body that you can enjoy for the entire day. You'll be calmly resting your attention on your breath to help get you in tune with yourself so you can deal with whatever the day brings your way with focus, grace, and ease.

Remember, it's important to practice with ease. How you practice matters more than what you practice. You can practice yoga tense, try to force your body into the poses while gritting your teeth and furrowing your brow, or you can allow your body to move with ease, allow your breath to be full and deep, and enjoy the ride. Your body and life will transform to reflect how you practice. Practice tense and you'll build more tension. Practice with ease and you'll get capable and be able to do more with less effort.

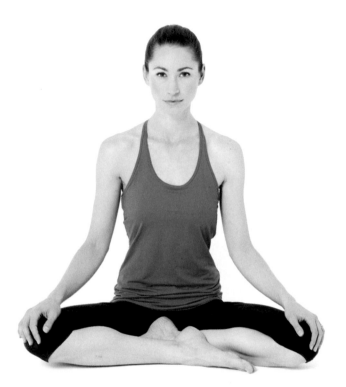

☆ EASY SEATED

Sit comfortably with your legs crossed and your back straight. If it doesn't feel okay to cross your legs, try sitting on your heels instead. Relax your hands on your thighs. Close your eyes and take a big inhale through your nose and then a long exhale through your mouth. Set a nice, deep pace of breathing you can stay with for a while. When you are ready, open your eyes.

EASY SEATED SIDE BEND

Relax your right hand on the ground on your right side. Soften your right elbow, arc your left arm up, and bend over your right side. Take a few big deep breaths here. When you are ready, roll back up to center and do the same on the other side.

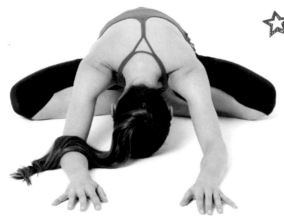

EASY SEATED FORWARD BEND

Walk your hands out in front of you until you feel a nice opening. It might be a few steps today, and perhaps a few more tomorrow. Don't worry about how far you can bend. Just go with how you feel. Allow your body to shift and drift along with your breath.

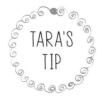

TARA'S TIP

EACH INHALE CREATES A LITTLE MORE ROOM INSIDE YOUR BODY AND MIND. EACH EXHALE MOVES YOU RIGHT INTO THAT NEW SPACE. THE DEEPER YOU BREATHE, THE MORE SPACE OPENS UP!

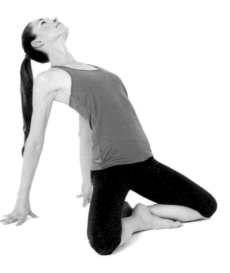

☆ EASY SEATED BACK ARCH

Press your fingertips behind you on the ground. Take a big inhale as you press down through your fingertips to lift your body up. As you exhale, gently lower your hips back to the ground and relax.

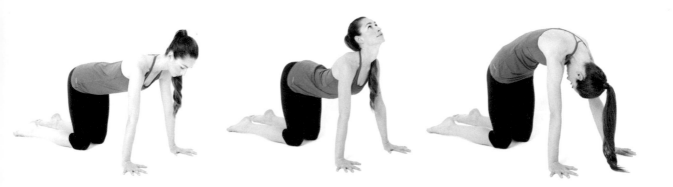

☆ ALL FOURS, COW, CAT

Shift your hips to one side and roll onto all fours. Take a big inhale as you drop your belly down toward the ground and look up (cow). As you exhale, round your back and look toward your stomach (cat). Allow your body to move how you feel.

DOWN DOG

Tuck your toes and take a big deep inhale to lift your hips up and back to down dog. Relax your head, neck, and shoulders. Allow your body to shift side to side or forward and back to open up. Hang here for five long, deep breaths.

DOWN DOG SPLIT

On a big inhale, lift your right leg up and back. Open your hips if that feels good to you. Feel free to bend your knee and roll your hips around a bit.

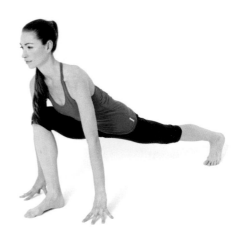

 ## LOW LUNGE

Step your right foot between your hands into a low lunge. If your foot doesn't make it on your first try, no worries; try grabbing your ankle with your right hand and giving it a nice gentle boost. Hang here for five long, deep breaths.

LOW LUNGE BACK KNEE DOWN ARCH

From your low lunge, ease your back knee down to the ground. Take a big inhale and open your chest up. If you feel good with your fingertips on the ground, keep them there. If it feels nicer to open your arms up and back, open on up!

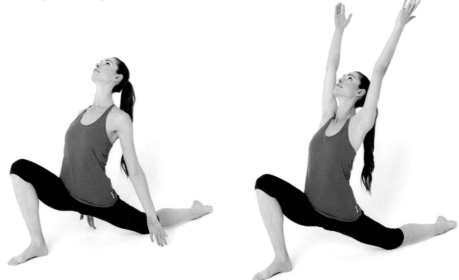

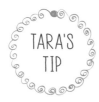 **TARA'S TIP**

THE GOAL IS TO CONNECT WITH YOURSELF AND FEEL GREAT, NOT TO DO YOGA POSES. FORGET ABOUT THE POSES AND ALLOW YOURSELF TO FEEL.

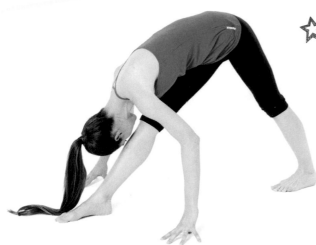

☆ SINGLE LEG FORWARD BEND

Press your fingertips on the ground on either side of your front foot. Take a big inhale and lift your hips up. Relax your torso over your front leg. If your legs don't straighten easily, bend your knees and roll around in your hips and torso a bit. Keep easy in your body and let your torso sway side to side. Hang here for five long, deep breaths.

☆ HIGH LUNGE

Exhale and sink back into your low lunge. Press firmly through your legs and take a big inhale as you lift your hips into a high lunge, with your arms straight above your head.

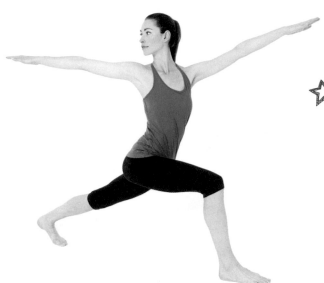

 ## ☆ HIGH LUNGE TWIST

As you exhale, twist to your right and open your arms out to your sides. As you inhale, come back into a high lunge. Try this twice more with your breath.

☆ WARRIOR 2

Exhale open to warrior 2. To do this, ground your back heel down, open your arms out to your sides, and sink your hips so your front knee is directly over your front ankle, not rolling in or out. Angle your back foot so your toes are pointing 45 degrees toward your front. You should feel a nice opening in your hips. Gaze over your front fingers. Hang here for five long, deep breaths.

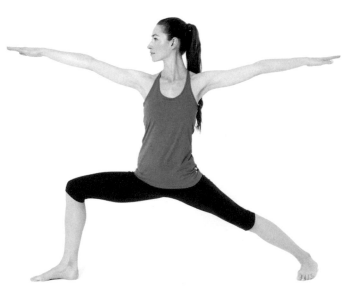

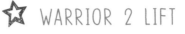

☆ WARRIOR 2 LIFT

From warrior 2, inhale as you lift your hips up, straightening your front leg, and extend your arms over your head. Exhale back to warrior 2. Repeat twice more.

☆ REVERSE WARRIOR

From warrior 2, inhale and tip your torso back. Let your left hand slide down your back leg. Arch your right arm up and over your head. Gaze upward if that feels good. If looking upward doesn't feel good on your neck, gaze down toward your left hand.

⭐ EXTENDED SIDE ANGLE

From reverse warrior, as you exhale, tip your torso up and over toward your front thigh. Rest your right forearm on your right thigh. Arch your left arm up and over your head. Gaze up toward your left palm if that feels good. If looking upward doesn't feel good on your neck, look straight out to your side, keeping your neck aligned on your spine.

⭐ WARRIOR 3

From extended side angle, bring your fingertips to the ground on either side of your front foot and come onto your back toes so you are in a low lunge. Keep your hips lifted high (to protect your knee) and crawl your fingertips out in front of you a few steps until you are standing on your right leg. Straighten your right leg, and lift your left leg up behind you, even with your hips. Flex your foot and point your toes toward the ground.

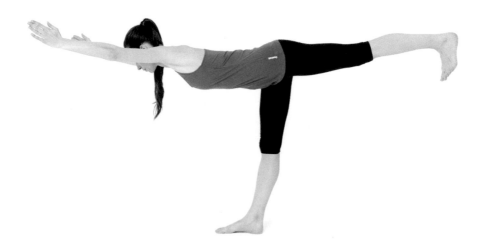

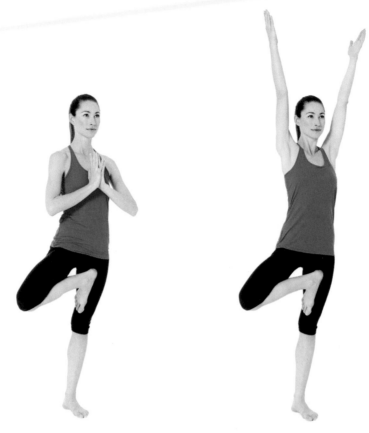

 TREE

From warrior 3, soften both knees, round your back, and roll up to stand, bringing your right leg along with you and hugging it into your chest with your arms. Place the bottom of your right foot into your left upper thigh and let your knee open out to your side. If that doesn't feel good, place your toes on the ground with the bottom of your foot connecting with your ankle. To keep the balance, press your foot into your thigh and your thigh into your foot, like a magnet to your fridge, equal pressure both ways. If you like, bring your palms together, thumbs at your chest, and lift your chest up. If you'd rather, extend your arms straight up. Relax your shoulders, your head, and your gaze.

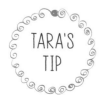

TARA'S TIP

THERE IS ALWAYS MOVEMENT IN BALANCE, SO MAKE SURE TO STAY EASY IN YOUR BODY SO YOU CAN ALLOW YOUR BODY TO DRIFT AND SHIFT IN THE BREEZE. IF TREES NEVER MOVED THEIR BRANCHES AND LEAVES, THEY WOULD BE STIFF AND FALL OVER. STRONG TREES ARE STURDY IN THEIR ROOTS AND MOVABLE IN THEIR BRANCHES.

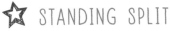 ## STANDING SPLIT

From tree, hug your shin
back into your chest with
your arms. Dive over
your standing (right) leg,
softening your knee until
your fingertips reach the
ground. Allow your left leg
to lift up behind you. Relax
your head and neck. Take
a few breaths to soften
through your standing leg
and roll your hips around
to open up any tight
spaces.

LOW LUNGE

Soften through both legs and step your left leg back to your low lunge. Place your fingertips on the ground on either side of your front foot for support. Sink your hips low. Reach out through your back heel and lift your back thigh up.

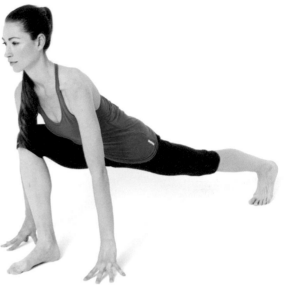

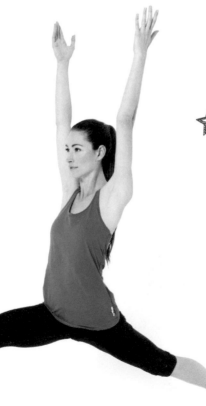

HIGH LUNGE

From low lunge, press firmly down through both legs, and on a big inhale lift your torso and arms up, so your shoulders are over your hips. Exhale and soften right where you are. Relax your head, neck, and shoulders. Extend out through your back heel and lift your back thigh up.

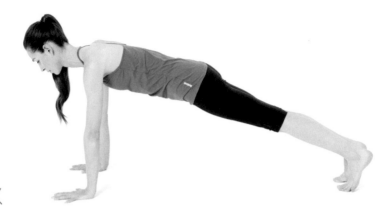

⭐ PLANK

Exhale your palms to the ground on either side of your front foot and step back into a plank position. Extend the top of your head forward and your heels back. Lift your belly and your thighs up, keeping your body in a straight line from your shoulders to your heels. Stay here for ten long, deep breaths.

⭐ SIDE PLANK

From plank, press into your right hand and roll to the outside edge of your right foot. Open your body to your left side, putting your arm straight up into the air. Either keep both feet on the ground, slightly apart for stability, or stack your feet on top of each other. Gaze either upward at your top hand or out to the side, whichever feels better on your neck. Stay here for three long, deep breaths.

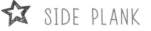

SIDE PLANK TREE

If you feel steady in your side plank, try lifting your top leg into tree pose, pressing the bottom of your foot either on the calf or above the knee of your bottom leg. Try not to press your foot directly on your knee, to keep your knees safe and happy. Stay here for three long, deep breaths.

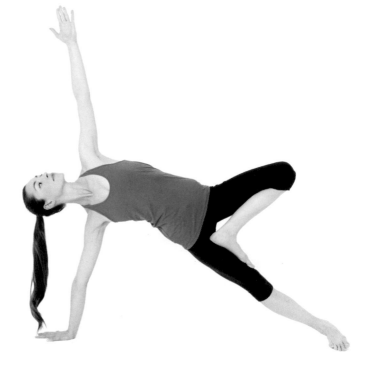

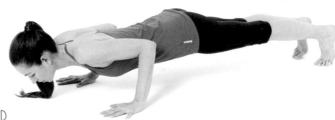

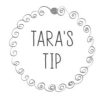 ## PUSH UP

Roll back into plank. Bend your elbows and lower your body halfway down to the floor. Press straight back up. Repeat twice more; the third time, lower all the way down onto your belly.

TARA'S TIP

TRY TO KEEP YOUR BODY IN ONE LINE AS YOU LOWER AND LIFT. IF YOU ARE DIPPING YOUR HIPS AND ARCHING YOUR BACK, PUT YOUR KNEES ON THE GROUND FOR EXTRA SUPPORT. THIS WILL SAVE YOUR BACK FROM PAIN OVER TIME.

UP DOG

Press your palms on the ground next to your chest and lift your torso up a bit, leaving your knees on the ground. Allow your torso to sway side to side as you come up. Roll your shoulders down your back, take a big inhale, and lift up to a place where it feels like you are getting a nice opening. If this doesn't feel good on your lower back, soften your elbows until your torso is a lot closer to the floor. When you are ready, relax back down to lie on your belly.

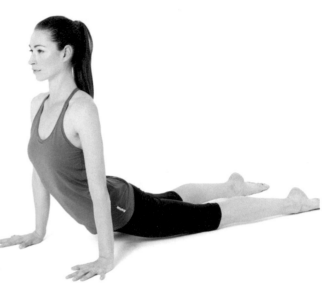

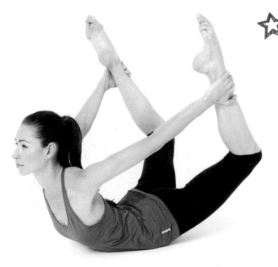

BOW

From lying on your belly, bend your knees, reach behind you, and grab your ankles. Gently press your feet into your hands to lift yourself up. Rock easily forward and back on your belly. Hang here for five long, deep breaths, then relax back down to lie on your belly. Rest for a few moments and repeat.

CHILD'S POSE

Shift your hips back to sit on your heels. Relax your arms out in front of you and rest your forehead on the ground. Allow your attention to draw deeper inward and let your body relax. Breathe deeply here until you feel ready to move on.

 ## SIT ON HEELS

Roll your torso up so you are sitting up on your heels. Relax your shoulders down your back, and rest your hands on your thighs with your palms down. Close your eyes and take a big deep inhale through your nose. Exhale out your mouth. Repeat twice more; then, when you are ready, gently open your eyes.

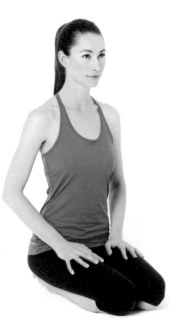

AFTER YOU'VE FINISHED THIS ROUTINE, GO BACK AND DO IT AGAIN,
BUT THIS TIME, USE THE OPPOSITE SIDE OF YOUR BODY.

You did it! Great job! I hope you are feeling energized, inspired, and ready to begin your day. If you have a moment, it might be useful to document your experience in a practice journal. Write down how you feel, any ideas that came up during your practice, and what was easy and challenging for you.

CRAVING CONTROL FLOW—SAY GOOD-BYE TO CRAVINGS AND FOOD ADDICTIONS

Experiencing cravings, food addictions, and a compulsion to binge are very real and scary issues to deal with on your own. Having a regular practice to deal with anxiety and compulsion is a great way to set your mind at ease and get your body back to a place where you feel good, strong, empowered, and in control. This routine is designed to get your body moving and calm your mind.

When cravings emerge, so does restless physical and mental anxiety. The breath work in this practice is designed to dissolve the tension so you can come back to an easygoing physical and mental state. The movements are designed to open up and calm the hips, hamstrings, shoulders, and spine, the major areas where we hold tension and stress when we experience cravings.

If you have problems with food anxiety and compulsion, try this routine in the morning and at night to ease your mind and balance your body. Also try the routine during the moments you experience anxiety and negative urges around food. If you have no problems with compulsion and anxiety around food, this routine is still great for calming your mind and keeping your body open and sensitized so you can listen to what it needs to be fueled properly.

If you are in the compulsion camp, let the guilt stop right here. I'm giving you a virtual hug right now and letting you know that you're going to be okay and there is nothing to be afraid of. With regular practice, you'll be feeling fantastic in no time. Just stick with yourself and you'll be on your way to greatness. We're in this together. Stay easy and be patient with yourself.

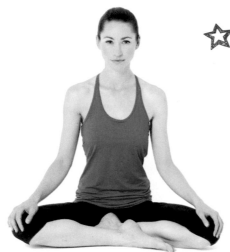

☆ EASY SEATED

Sit comfortably with your legs crossed and your back straight. If it doesn't feel okay to cross your legs, try sitting on your heels instead. Relax your hands on your thighs. Close your eyes and take a big inhale through your nose and long exhale out through your mouth. Set a nice, deep pace of breathing you can stay with for a while. When you are ready, open your eyes.

☆ ARMS IN V

From your easy seated position, extend your arms up so they are in a V shape. Relax your shoulders, head, neck, and face. Relax your entire body, while you keep your arms up. We'll stay here for three minutes. Feel free to set a timer, use a watch, or simply count deep breaths. When you're finished, relax your arms down by your sides.

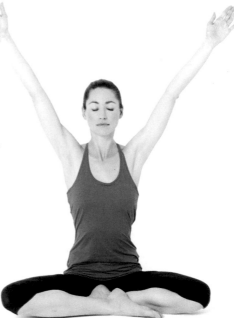

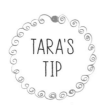

TARA'S TIP

NOTICE SENSATIONS WITHOUT REACTING. WHEN YOUR ARMS ARE UP FOR THREE MINUTES, THEY WILL START TO FEEL DIFFERENT FROM WHEN THEY WERE RESTING DOWN. KNOW THEY AREN'T GOING TO FALL OFF. NOTHING BAD WILL HAPPEN. SIMPLY STAY AND OBSERVE. ALLOW YOUR BODY AND MIND TO RELAX WHILE YOU ARE WORKING. FIND THE LEAST AMOUNT OF EFFORT YOU CAN USE TO STAY HERE.

SEATED SINGLE LEG EXTEND SIDE BEND

From easy seated, open your right leg out toward your right side. Relax your right arm on the ground inside your right leg. Soften your elbow and lean to your right side. On a big inhale, arc your left arm up and over your head. When you are ready, gently come back to sitting upright.

SEATED SINGLE LEG EXTEND EASY TWIST

Place your right hand on your left upper thigh and your left fingertips on the ground alongside your spine. Inhale and lift your torso. Exhale and twist around easily to your left side. Switch legs and do the other side.

☆ SEATED STRADDLE

Open both legs out to the side. Press your
hands into the ground behind your legs, lift
your hips, and scoot yourself forward or back,
however it feels nice to get a good opening.
Either stay upright or relax your torso forward,
depending on how you feel. Make sure you
can breathe easily and fully.

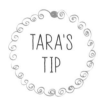

DEEP BREATHS ARE TENSION'S KRYPTONITE. KEEP ON
BREATHING DEEP!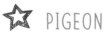

☆ PIGEON

Bend your right knee and angle your shin so it is facing
your front. Bring your left leg around behind you and
extend it. If there's pain or tension in your right knee,
scootch your right foot closer toward your body. Move
your hips around until you feel a nice opening. If you feel
great sitting upright, stay there. If you'd like to walk your
hands out forward and relax your torso, that version is a
great opening, too. Feel free to crawl around from side to
side exploring all your parts.

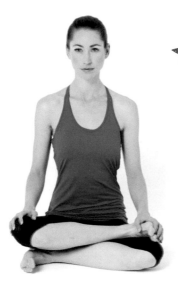

☆ ANKLE TO KNEE

Bring your back leg around and stack your front leg on top of it, ankles and shins on top of each other. If that hurts or doesn't feel easy, slide your left leg in front of your right for an easy seated position. Bring your fingertips behind you on the ground and lean back. Either stay here if this feels like a nice opening or bring your hands in front of you and walk your torso forward.

☆ COW FACE

Stack your knees on top of each other (right on top of left) and let your feet rest out to your sides. If this doesn't feel good on your knees, don't push or force your body into the shape, just stay in easy seated for a few more breaths. If you are comfortable with your knees stacked, take a few breaths here. You can either stay upright or rest your torso forward. When you are finished, bring your torso upright.

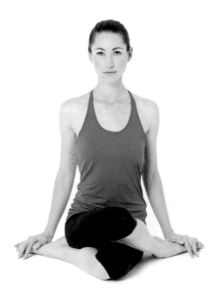

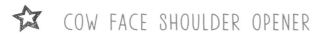

COW FACE SHOULDER OPENER

Lift your left arm overhead, bend your elbow, and relax your arm down your back. Bend your right elbow and slide your right arm up your back. If your hands find each other easily, hook them together; if not, leave some space between your hands. Either stay upright or relax your torso forward over your legs.

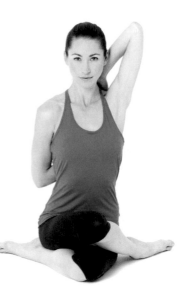

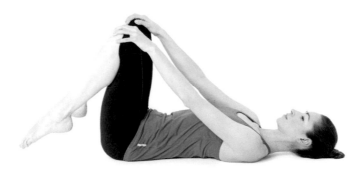

RECLINING BOTH KNEES HUG

Bring your arms back to your sides and gently roll down on your back. Hug your knees into your chest and rock easily side to side to release any tension in your back and hips.

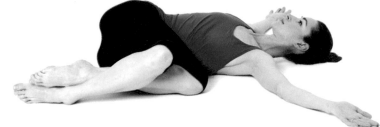

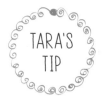

⭐ RECLINING EAGLE TWIST

Place the soles of your feet flat on the ground beneath your hips. Lift your hips up and scoot them over to your right side. Wrap your right leg around your left leg and let your knees relax over to your left side. Open your arms out to your sides and look over toward your right hand.

TARA'S TIP

MAKE YOUR OWN RULES AS YOU FEEL INTO THE FULL RANGE OF YOURSELF. YOU'LL GET SO MUCH MORE OUT OF YOUR PRACTICE IF YOU ALLOW YOURSELF TO FEEL RATHER THAN JUST GOING THROUGH THE POSES.

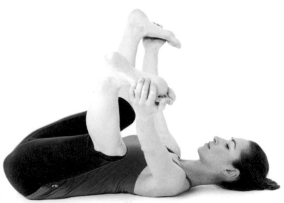

⭐ HAPPY BABY

Come back to lying on your back, and then hug your knees into your chest. Bring the bottoms of your feet to point upward, so your knees are at a 90-degree angle. Grab the outside of each foot with your hands and gently draw your knees toward the ground outside your hips. Rock side to side, however feels good to you.

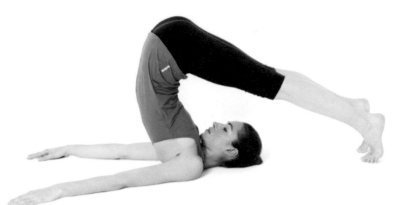

⭐ PLOW

If your back feels okay, roll your feet up and over your head. Soften your knees as you roll up and over. If your neck doesn't feel good here, roll down and relax. Don't worry about pushing your toes to the ground if they don't reach naturally. Stay wherever you feel good.

⭐ SHOULDER STAND

If you feel good in plow, press the palms of your hands into the small of your back for support, fingers facing up. Then allow your legs to float and lift up, pointing your toes toward the ceiling. Gaze toward your belly button.

When you are ready to come out of shoulder stand, ease your feet back over your head. Soften your knees a bit. Relax your arms down by your sides and slowly roll down to lie on your back. Keep your knees bent as you roll down to be easy on your back.

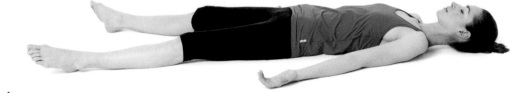

☆ RELAXATION

When you are ready, lie down to relax. Open your legs and arms a bit to your sides. Close your eyes. Take a big inhale through your nose. Exhale out through your mouth. Repeat this twice more. Return to normal breathing through your nose.

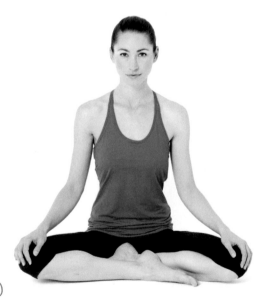

☆ EASY SEATED

From relaxation, start to bring a little more air back into your body. Move your fingers and toes around. Interlace your hands and take a nice stretch over your head. Hug your knees into your chest and rock up to sit up tall. Roll around a bit in your body until you find a nice, neutral balanced point. Close your eyes and take a few big deep breaths. When you are ready, open your eyes.

ONCE YOU'VE FINISHED, HEAD BACK TO THE BEGINNING
AND WORK THE MOVES WITH THE OPPOSITE SIDE OF YOUR BODY.

Great job! I hope you feel calm, connected, and easy in your body. Make sure to practice every day, if only for a few moments. Your body and mind will thank you!

BODY AWARENESS FLOW—BRINGING ATTENTION TO EVERY PART OF YOU

One of the aims of regular practice is to build body awareness. When we are anxious, stressed, and not practicing regularly, we're likely not paying attention to where we are in space. Sensitizing your body and mind to how you feel is an invaluable skill that will enhance your quality of life. Knowing what your body and mind need through feeling, rather than thinking or seeking outside approval, is incredibly empowering. Being sensitized is like being in control of what you need when you need it. Gone are the days of insecurity, second-guessing yourself, and searching for the right thing to do. When you are sensitized, you are connected to how you feel from the inside, and it's easy to follow up with the actions that keep you connected to feeling.

I designed this routine to sensitize every part of your body. When you have good body awareness, you are in touch with how you feel and what your body needs to be ridiculously healthy and happy. We'll go a little slower than usual in this routine so you can take the time to feel into all your parts. The movements will build strength in your entire body and allow your mind to be calm and focused. Don't rush through the movements. Stay easy in your body; remember to breathe deeply and have a great time!

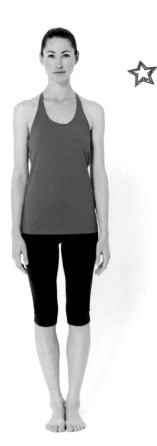

STANDING

Start standing up nice and tall with your arms hanging at your sides. Bring your feet parallel to each other and a little bit apart. Close your eyes and relax your body. Soften your knees. Relax your head, neck, and shoulders. Allow yourself to shift and drift side to side and forward and back. Stay here for five long, deep breaths, and when you are ready, open your eyes.

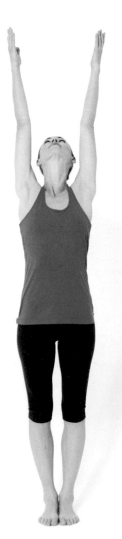

STANDING ARM REACH

Inhale and reach your arms out and all the way up above your head. Lengthen through your sides and gaze upward.

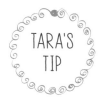

TARA'S TIP

YOU ARE A SPACE MAKER. AS YOU INHALE, FILL UP ALL THE SPACE AROUND YOU. AS YOU EXHALE, SOFTEN AND RELAX. FEEL THE NICE SENSE OF CALM IN YOUR BODY AND MIND.

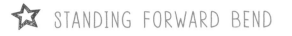

⭐ STANDING FORWARD BEND

As you exhale, gently roll your torso over your legs. Bend your knees to take the pressure out of your hamstrings. Allow your torso to sway gently side to side, lingering where it feels nice to linger. Let your head and neck relax.

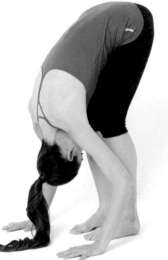

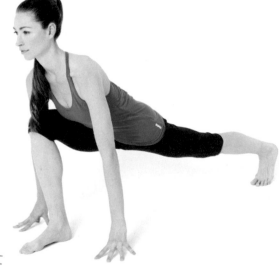

⭐ LOW LUNGE

Soften your knees, press your fingertips on the ground, and step your left leg back to a low lunge. Sink your hips low and rock side to side. Extend out through your back heel and lengthen out through the top of your head. Hang here moving easily for five long, deep breaths.

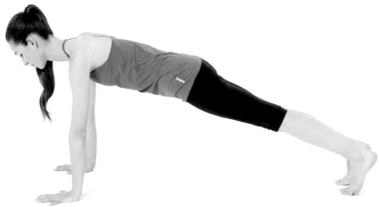

☆ PLANK

Press your palms firmly on the ground on either side of your front foot and step back to plank. Lengthen the top of your head forward and extend your heels back behind you. Lift your belly and your thighs up, keeping your body in a straight line from your head to your heels.

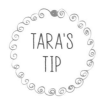

TARA'S TIP IF YOU FEEL YOUR BODY OR MIND GETTING STIFF OR TENSE, MOVE A BIT, SWAYING A LITTLE SIDE TO SIDE TO KEEP THE EASE.

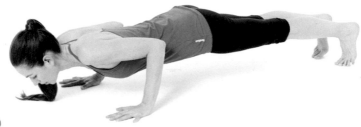

☆ PUSH UP

Bend your elbows alongside your ribs. Exhale as you lower your body half-way down. You can do this with your knees lifted or on the floor—your call. Inhale and press straight back up. Repeat twice more; the third time lower all the way down onto your belly.

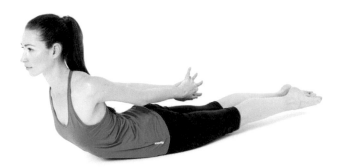

☆ LYING ON BELLY BACK OPENER

From lying on your belly, interlace your hands behind your back, palms facing one another, and lift your chest and legs up. Extend the top of your head forward, keeping the back of your neck nice and long. Extend your legs behind you. Roll side to side on your belly to keep everything soft and open. When you are ready, relax back down to your belly.

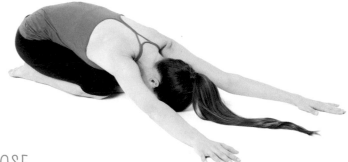

☆ CHILD'S POSE

From lying on your belly, plant your palms on the ground on either side of your chest. Shift your hips to sit on your heels. Relax your forehead on the ground. Allow your body to shift and drift from side to side. Stay here for five long, deep breaths.

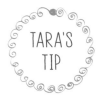

TARA'S TIP

ALLOW YOUR BODY TO MOVE AND LINGER WHERE IT FEELS NICE TO LINGER. MOVEMENT IS A GOOD THING. IT HELPS YOU FEEL INTO ALL YOUR PARTS.

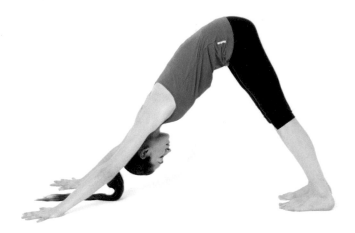

 ## DOWN DOG

From child's pose, shift onto all fours. Roll around in your spine a bit. Let your breath move your body. Linger where it feels nice to linger. When you are ready, tuck your toes, take a big inhale, and lift your hips up and back to down dog. Pedal through your feet and shift your weight around to feel into all your parts. When you are ready, walk your feet up toward your hands. Don't worry about keeping your hands anchored in place—they can walk forward, too.

 ## STANDING FORWARD BEND

Step your feet parallel to each other, a little bit apart. Hang your torso over your legs. If your hamstrings feel tight, bend your knees and rest your torso on your legs. Let your head and neck relax. Allow your body to sway from side to side.

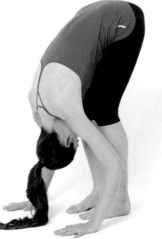

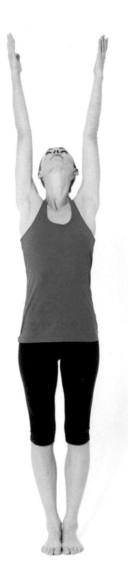

☆ STANDING ARM REACH

From standing forward bend, on a big inhale, gently roll up to stand and reach your arms out and up over your head. Exhale and relax your arms down by your sides.

REPEAT THE ROUTINE ON THE OPPOSITE SIDE.
STAY EASY AND ENJOY THE RIDE!

EASY MIND CALM BODY FLOW—FIND THE EASE FROM THE INSIDE OUT

This is a superquick routine you can practice anytime of day to bring your body and mind back to restful, open ease. If you are feeling tense, tight, or stressed, find some open space and breathe through this easygoing flow to release anything you don't need. You can use this even if you have only a few minutes. You'll be amazed what a little movement can do to calm you.

This routine was designed to open up your sides and spine, create room in your entire body, and calm your mind. Stay easy as you move through the routine and allow your body and mind to settle as you move gently with your breath. Not only will this calm you from the inside out, it'll allow you to be more energized and focused, so you can move on with your day, your project, or even your relaxation time from a better place.

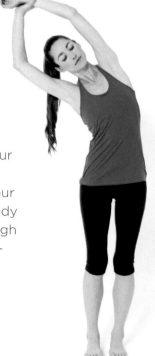

 ## STANDING SIDE BEND

Start standing nice and tall. Inhale and reach your arms out and up over your head. Grab your left wrist with your right hand. Exhale and soften your knees and shoulders. Inhale and stretch your body up and over toward your right side. Come through center, exhale, and soften your knees and shoulders; then inhale and stretch your body up and over toward your left side.

STANDING FORWARD BEND WRIST RELEASE

From standing, roll your torso down over your legs. Soften your knees as you go. Bend your knees enough so you can step on your hands. Relax your head, neck, and shoulders.

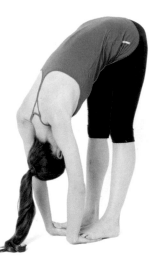

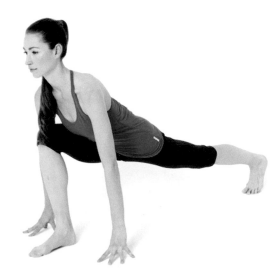

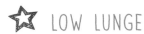

LOW LUNGE

Remove your hands from under your feet. Press your fingertips on the ground, bend your knees, and step your left leg back into a low lunge. Sink your hips and allow your body to sway side to side and forward and back, however feels good.

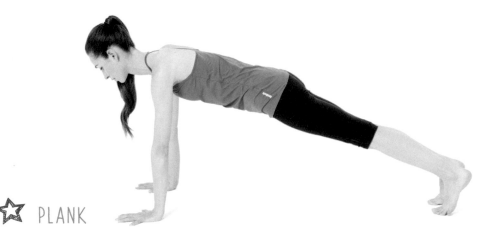

 ## PLANK

Plant your palms on the ground and step back to plank. Lengthen the top of your head forward and extend your heels back behind you. Lift your belly and your thighs up, keeping your body in a straight line from your head to your heels.

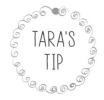 **TARA'S TIP** NO PAIN, LOTS OF GAIN. IF SOMETHING HURTS, THAT'S A GOOD SIGN TO BACK OFF. DON'T PUSH THROUGH PAIN, ESPECIALLY IN THE JOINTS.

 ## UP DOG

From plank, ease your knees down to the ground, soften your elbows, and open your chest forward into up dog. Allow your torso to sway from side to side. Roll your shoulders down your back, take a big inhale, and lift up to a place where it feels like you are getting a nice opening. If this doesn't feel good on your lower back, soften your elbows until your torso is a lot closer to the floor.

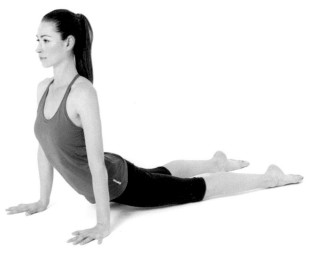

⭐ CHILD'S POSE

From up dog, keeping your knees on the ground, sink your hips to your heels and relax your forehead on the ground. Extend your arms forward. Stay here for five long, deep breaths.

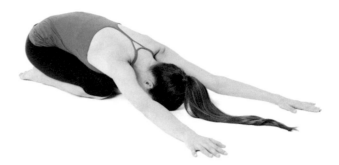

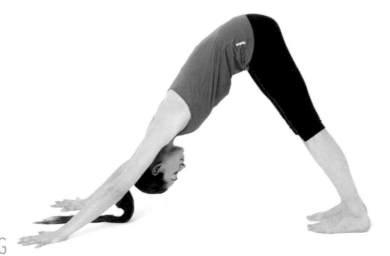

⭐ DOWN DOG

From child's pose, come onto all fours, tuck your toes, and lift your hips up and back to down dog. Relax your shoulders, head, and neck. Move your body how it feels good to move. Stay here for five long, deep breaths.

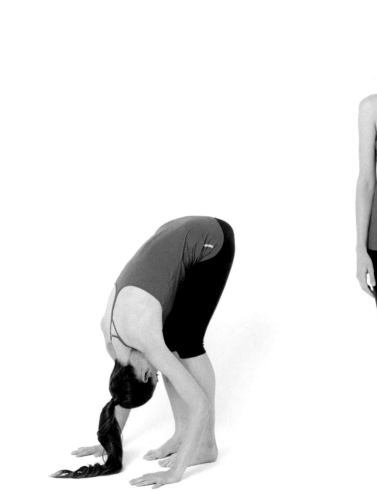

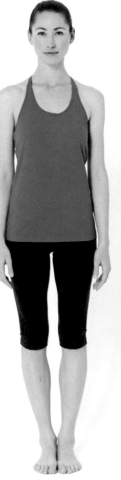

☆ STAND

Walk your feet up to your hands and fold forward for a few breaths. Slowly roll up to stand and repeat the entire routine on the other side. Roll through the entire routine four more times.

I hope you feel open and free after moving with ease in that flow. Try this routine a few times a week to get your calm on in a major way. Linger where it feels nice to linger and enjoy the ride!

HEART-PUMPING SWEATY FLOW—GAIN STRENGTH FROM THE INSIDE OUT

All this talk about moving with ease, cultivating body awareness, and settling anxiety doesn't mean that you're going to be only doing minimal movement and a physically easy practice. Just because you move with ease doesn't mean it's easy or you need to be lazy in the practice. Going after a calorie burn in a typical spin class or gym workout is one way to get your heart pumping and a good sweat on, but, as I'll continue to remind you, working out, when done with aggression, only adds more tension in your body and mind. This often results in a frazzled state, overeating, and continuing the cycle of binge and burn. Believe it or not, you can work up a giant heart-pumping sweat and keep a relaxed face the entire time if you approach yoga in an easygoing way. When you learn how to relax while you are working hard, you start to build a capable body and focused mind.

The neat thing about moving easily in yoga when it comes to strength-building, sweat-inducing exercise is that you are going to get the workout by simply doing the movements. There is no need to flex when you don't need to flex. There is no need to push harder when you don't need to push. Efficiency becomes the way of moving, and the result is a capable body and mind. When the goal isn't to "feel the burn," the practice becomes enjoyable. The goal is to sensitize and feel good. Working your body actually feels great when you allow yourself to be easy and to feel.

This practice cultivates a superhero strong body from the inside out. You're going to sweat, so get ready. The best way to build full-body strength and mobility is by working your entire body all at once in many different ways. So that's what we're going to do. This is going to be a fun adventure. Stay with it, and see you on the other side!

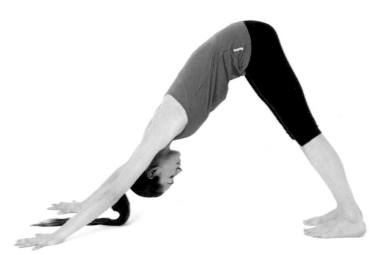

 DOWN DOG

Come onto all fours. Move your spine with your breath a bit to start to open up your body. When you are ready, tuck your toes, take a big inhale, and lift your hips up and back to down dog. Pedal through your feet and shift your weight around to feel into all your parts.

 DOWN DOG SPLIT

From down dog, take a big in-hale and lift your right leg back and up. Open your hips, bend your knee, and roll your hip and your ankle around in any way that feels good.

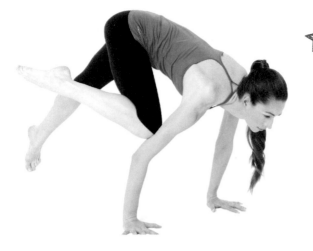

☆ KNEE HOVER

From down dog split, exhale and draw your right knee up and around to your right upper arm. Press your knee into the back of your upper arm and hover here. If you feel like going further, move into flying crow; if not, skip this step.

☆ FLYING CROW

When you bring your knee to your upper arm, look forward and lift your hips and belly up. Play around with the balance. If you feel steady, rock forward, lift up, and transfer your weight into your arms—your back leg might just float off the ground.

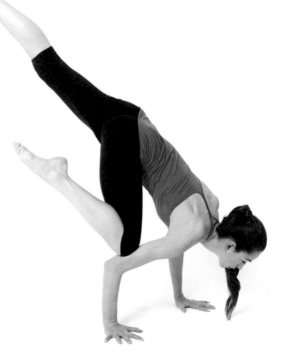

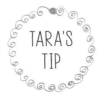

TARA'S TIP

DON'T JUMP OR FORCE YOUR WAY INTO ANYTHING. IT'S FUN TO TRY AND TO WORK ON, BUT REMEMBER, THE GOAL ISN'T TO DO POSES; IT'S TO BECOME INTUITIVE, CENTERED, CALM, AND CONNECTED. HAVE FUN WITH THIS ONE!

⭐ DOWN DOG SPLIT

From your knee hover or your flying crow, inhale and lift your leg back to down dog split.

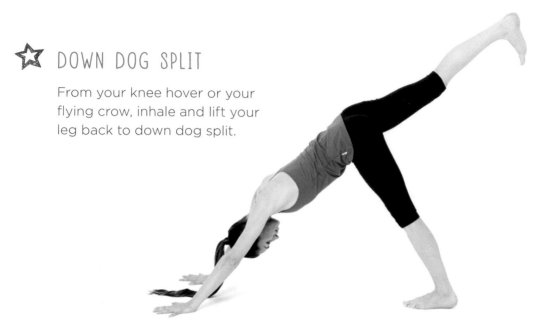

⭐ KNEE ACROSS

From down dog split, exhale and draw your knee across your body, pressing it into the back of your left upper arm. Bend your elbows slightly and make a shelf for your leg on your arm. Look forward and lean forward. If you feel like going further, move into twisted crow; if not, skip this step.

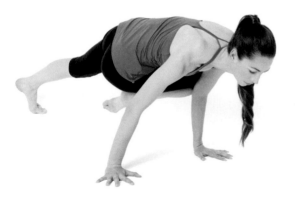

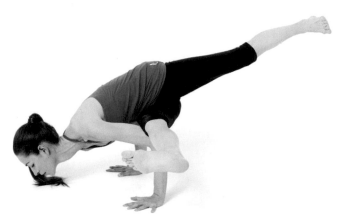

✩ TWISTED CROW

When you bring your knee across, make a shelf for your leg on your arm.
Lean forward, look forward, and lift your hips and belly up. If you feel
steady, rock forward enough to transfer your weight onto your arms and
play around with opening your legs out to the side.

✩ DOWN DOG SPLIT

From your knee across or twisted
crow, inhale and lift your leg back
and up to down dog split.

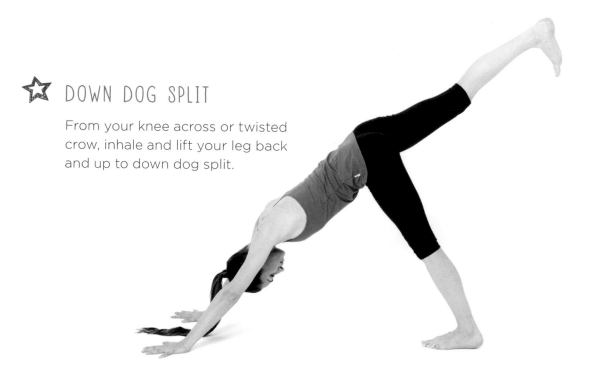

☆ LOW LUNGE

From down dog split, exhale and step your right leg forward to a low lunge. Come up on your fingertips and sink your hips low.

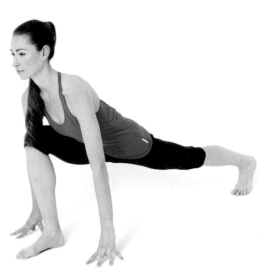

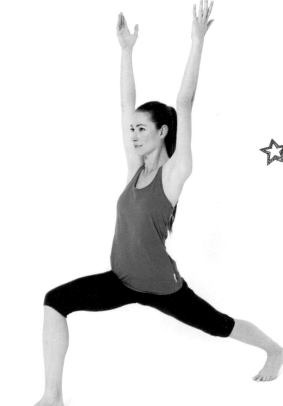

☆ HIGH LUNGE

From your low lunge, inhale and lift your hips and raise your arms above your head into a high lunge. Relax your shoulders down your back and extend out through your back heel.

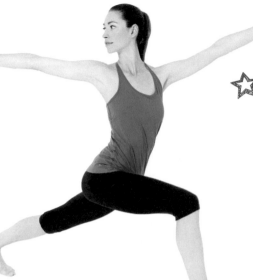

☆ HIGH LUNGE TWIST

From your high lunge, exhale and twist your torso toward your right side. Open your arms out to your sides and gaze to the side. Extend out through both arms evenly.

 ## HIGH LUNGE TWIST REVERSE

From high lunge twist, tip your torso back toward your back leg. Slide your right hand down your leg and float your left arm up. Gaze toward your bottom hand.

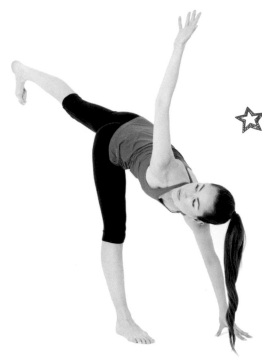

⭐ TWISTED HALF-MOON

From high lunge twist reverse, shift your weight forward onto your right leg, lifting your left leg up to be parallel to the ground. Bring your left fingertips to the ground under your left shoulder. Soften your knees and twist your body to the right side, extending your right arm straight into the air. Inhale and open to your right side. Look up toward your right hand if it feels okay in your neck.

⭐ HALF-MOON

From twisted half-moon, place your right finger-tips on the ground under your right shoulder, keeping your left leg up. Open your body to your left side and extend your left arm up. Gaze up toward your left hand if it feels okay in your neck.

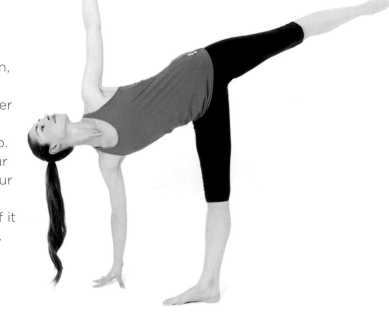

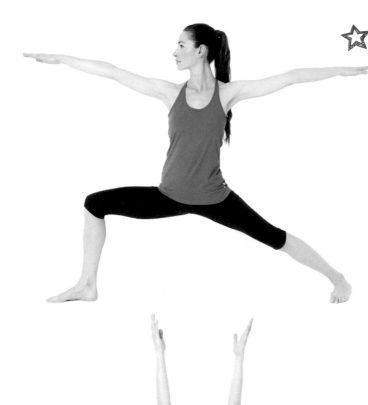

⭐ WARRIOR 2

Soften your knees, and step your left foot back a few feet so both of your feet are on the ground. Inhale and lift your arms and hips up, straightening your front leg and extending your arms above your head. Exhale and sink into warrior 2. Point your front foot forward and turn your back toes slightly in. Sink your hips and bend your front knee so your knee is over your front ankle. Extend your arms out to your sides, and gaze over your front hand.

⭐ WARRIOR 2 LIFT

From warrior 2, inhale as you lift your hips up, straightening your front leg, and extend your arms over your head. Exhale back to warrior 2. Repeat twice more.

☆ REVERSE WARRIOR

From warrior 2, inhale and tip your torso back and slide your left arm down your left leg. Reach your right arm over your head and gaze up toward your right hand.

☆ EXTENDED SIDE ANGLE

From reverse warrior, exhale and bring your torso toward your front leg. Press your right forearm on your right thigh and extend your left arm up and over your head, lengthening through your left side. Gaze up toward your left hand.

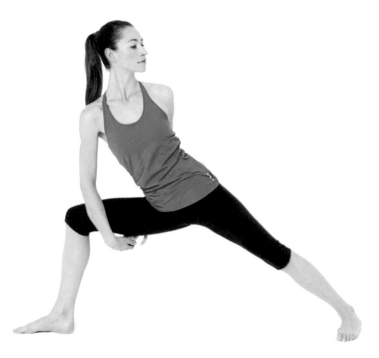

⭐ EXTENDED SIDE ANGLE WRAP

Wrap your top arm around your back. If it's easy for you, bring your bottom hand under your right upper thigh and interlace your hands. If the wrap won't happen without forcing or pushing, don't worry about it—just stay in extended side angle.

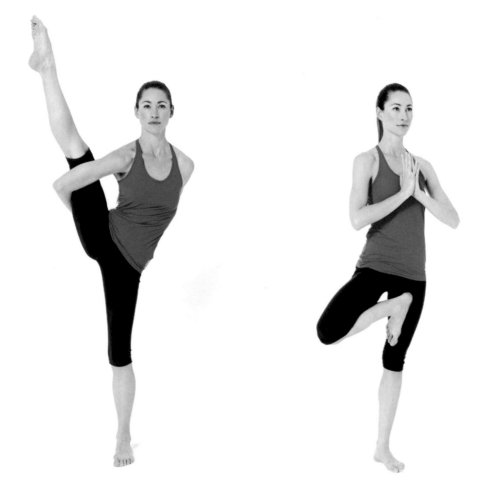

⭐ BIRD OF PARADISE OR TREE

If you are in extended side angle wrap, step your back foot forward to meet your front foot. Transfer your weight onto your left leg, and, keeping your arms around your upper thigh, extend your right leg out to the side if there is space in your body.

If you are in extended side angle, step your back foot forward to meet your front foot. Transfer your weight onto your left leg, and come up onto your left leg, holding your right shin with your right hand. Open your hip out to the side and press the bottom of your foot into your upper thigh.

If neither of these options feels good, simple place your toes on the ground with the bottom of your right foot connecting with your left ankle.

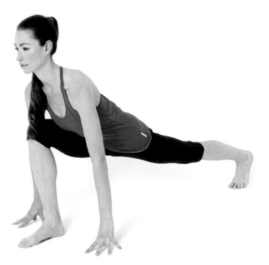

⭐ EXTENDED SIDE ANGLE

With control, bring your right foot to the ground next to your left. Unwrap your arms (if they are wrapped) and gently step back to extended side angle.

⭐ LOW LUNGE

Bring your fingertips to the ground on either side of your front foot. Come onto your back toes and sink your hips low.

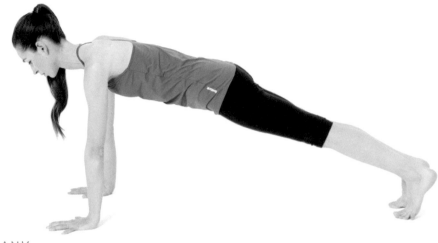

 ## PLANK

Plant your palms on the ground and step back to plank. Extend the top of your head forward and your heels back. Lift your belly and thighs up, keeping your body in a straight line from your head to your heels.

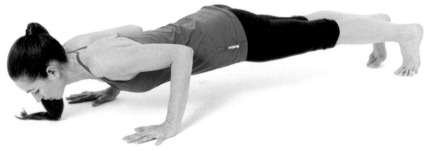

 ## PUSH UP

From plank, bend your elbows as you exhale and lower your body halfway down so your torso brushes alongside your upper arms. Inhale and press back up to plank. Repeat twice more.

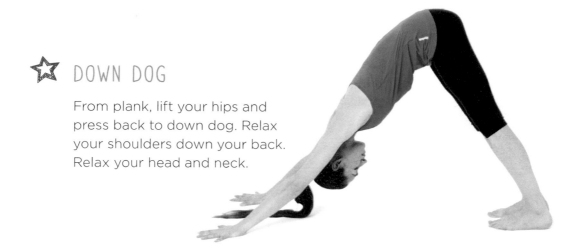

☆ DOWN DOG

From plank, lift your hips and press back to down dog. Relax your shoulders down your back. Relax your head and neck.

REPEAT THIS SEQUENCE FROM THE BEGINNING, FOCUSING ON THE LEFT SIDE, BEFORE YOU MOVE INTO THE NEXT PART OF THE ROUTINE.

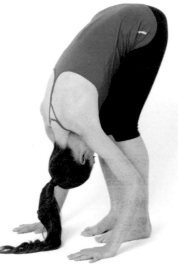

STANDING FORWARD BEND

From down dog, walk your feet up to your hands and fold your torso over your legs. Soften your knees to relax your hamstrings. Sway your torso from side to side.

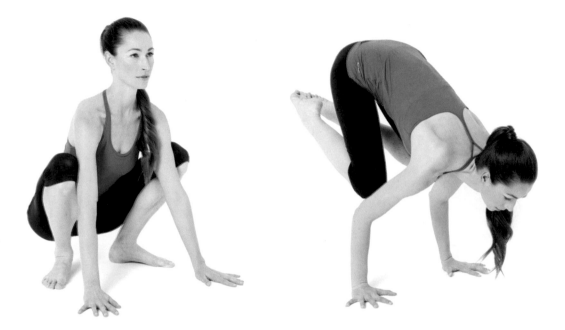

 ## CROW

Press your palms into the ground and bend your knees to come into a squat. Plant your palms about a foot in front of your toes. Inhale and rock forward. Press your knees into the backs of your upper arms. Lift your hips and belly up. Look forward. Keep your toes on the ground. Exhale and rock back to squat. Try a few more times. Maybe one toe comes off the ground the next time. Maybe the time after that the other toe comes off the ground. Maybe the time after that both toes come off the ground. Soon you'll be balancing completely on your arms.

TARA'S TIP

LOOK INTO THE FUTURE. MY FAVORITE CROW POSE TIP IS TO LOOK FORWARD. IF YOU LOOK DOWN, YOU'LL GO DOWN. IF YOU LOOK FORWARD, INTO THE FUTURE, ABOUT A FOOT IN FRONT OF YOU, YOU'LL LIFT UP AND GO FORWARD. HAVE FUN!

BOAT

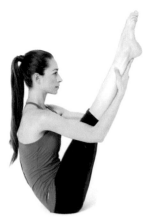

From crow, roll down to put your feet down.
Place your fingertips behind you on the ground
and gently ease yourself to sit on your hips with
your legs straight in front of you. Lift your legs
up and lengthen your spine, keeping your hands
raised up by your knees. If this is too much on
your lower back, bring your hands on the ground
behind you for support.

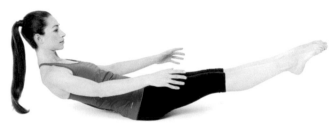

LOW BOAT

From boat, exhale and lower your body halfway down so your lower back is
on the ground, feet extended forward and head extended back. Inhale back
up to boat. Repeat lowering and lifting nine more times.

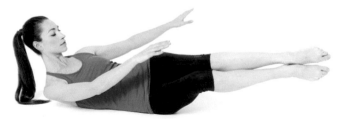

 BOAT TWIST

Exhale and roll onto your right hip and lower halfway down so your feet are
extended forward and your head extended back. Inhale back to boat. Exhale
and roll onto your left side. Inhale back to boat. Repeat nine more times.

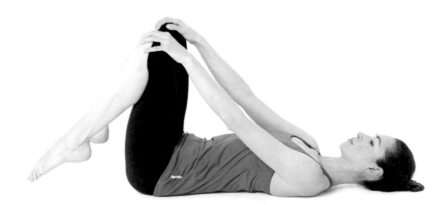

☆ RECLINING HUG KNEES

Exhale and lower halfway down to low boat. Hang here for three long, deep breaths. Relax all the way down onto your back and hug your knees into your chest. Rock side to side to release your lower back.

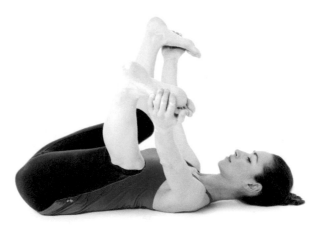

HAPPY BABY

Bring the bottoms of your feet to face up toward the ceiling. Grab the outside edge of each foot with your hands. Gently guide your legs closer to the ground. Rock side to side to open your hips and release your back.

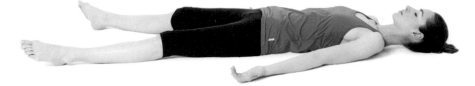

⭐ RELAXATION

From happy baby, when you feel ready, stretch out your arms and legs and lie down. Take a big inhale through your nose. Exhale out through your mouth. Repeat twice more. Close your eyes and relax.

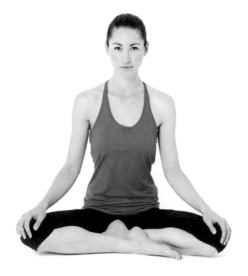

⭐ EASY SEATED

When you are ready, start to invite some more air back into your body. Roll your fingers and toes around to bring some attention into your body. Interlace your hands and take a nice stretch above your head and through your sides. Gently hug your knees into your chest and either rock onto your right side and rest there for a moment, or rock straight up to sit in easy seated pose. Relax your hands, palms down, on your thighs and allow your body to shift and drift side to side and forward and back with an aim of finding a neutral, balanced place. Allow your attention to drift right back inward.

I hope you feel great after that sweaty heart-pumping flow. Try this routine a few times a week to get you in your yoga groove, big-time. Stay easy, and remember to have fun!

EASYGOING WINDING DOWN
THE EVENING FLOW

Often when you're having trouble relaxing at the end of the day, it's anxiety that's keeping you up. It's coming from somewhere. No need to get stuck in your head about what you're not happy with in your life, and no need to feel bad about yourself at all. The beauty of regular easygoing yoga practice is that the anxiety, emotion, and psychology of whatever it is you are going through can work its way through and out of your system with the movement. Remember, it's not just exercise; it's physical, mental, and emotional maintenance. Without proper attention to all the aspects of who we are, we get out of balance and anxiety rushes in. We all need maintenance, and your regular practice is just the ticket to keep you healthy, calm, and connected.

I designed this practice to unwind any remaining tension in your body and mind that may be bundled and lurking around from a long day. We'll loosen up the shoulders, hips, hamstrings, back, and spine to let the stress out. Once the tension has released, you are free to enjoy a restful, rejuvenating sleep.

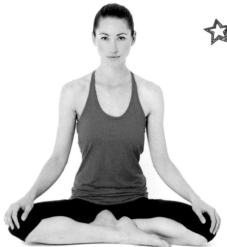

☆ EASY SEATED

Sit comfortably with your legs crossed and your back straight. If it doesn't feel okay to cross your legs, try sitting on your heels instead. Relax your hands on your thighs. Close your eyes and take a big inhale through your nose, then a long exhale through your mouth. Repeat twice more. Resume breathing in through your nose and out through your nose. Set a nice, big, full, deep pace of breath you can stay with for a while.

☆ EASY SEATED SIDE BEND

Relax your right hand on the ground on your right side. Soften your right elbow, arc your left arm up, and bend over your right side. Take a few big deep breaths here. When you are ready, roll back up to center and do the same on the other side, and then come back to center.

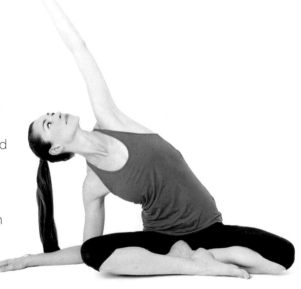

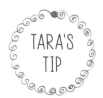

TARA'S
TIP

TENSION AND ANXIETY SEEP INTO YOUR BODY. IT'S PART OF LIFE. REGU-
LAR EASYGOING PRACTICE SENDS IT ON ITS WAY.

SEATED EASY TWIST

Inhale and lift your right arm out and up. Press your right hand on your left thigh. Press your left fingertips on the ground behind your spine. Exhale and twist to your left. Inhale and lift your torso upward. Exhale and twist a little farther around.

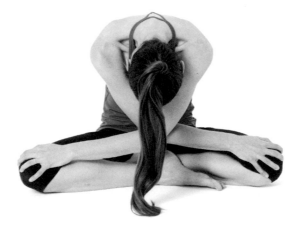

 ## SEATED OPPOSITE KNEE HOLD BACK RELEASE

Inhale and circle your left arm up over your head and across to your right thigh. Relax your torso forward. Relax your head and neck. When you are ready, release your hands and roll up to sit. Repeat on the other side from the seated easy twist.

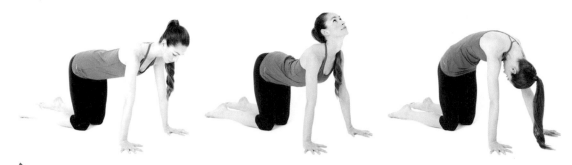

 ALL FOURS, COW, CAT

From easy seated, shift your weight to one side and come onto all fours. Spread your fingers wide like you are digging into sand. Inhale, drop your belly toward the ground, and look upward (cow). Exhale, round your back up, and look inward toward your belly (cat).

TARA'S TIP

THE DEEPER YOU BREATHE, THE MORE SPACE OPENS UP, SO BREATHE DEEP!

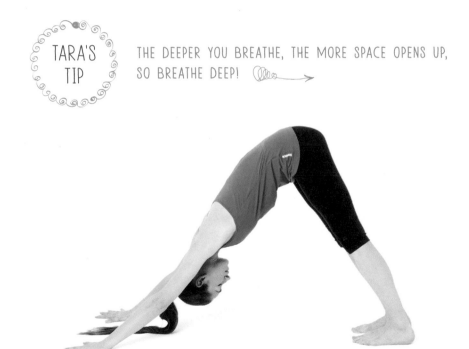

 DOWN DOG

From all fours, when you are ready, tuck your toes, take a big inhale, and lift your hips up and back to down dog. Pedal through your feet and shift your weight around to feel into all your parts.

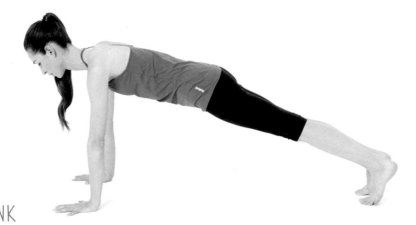

 ## PLANK

Tuck your chin in toward your chest and round your back to move into plank. Extend the top of your head forward and your heels back. Lift your belly and thighs up, keeping your body in a straight line from your head to your heels.

SIDE PLANK

From plank, press into your right hand and roll to the outside edge of your right foot. Open your body to your left side, putting your arm straight up into the air. Either keep both feet on the ground, slightly apart for stability, or stack your feet on top of each other. Gaze either upward at your top hand or out to the side, whichever feels better on your neck.

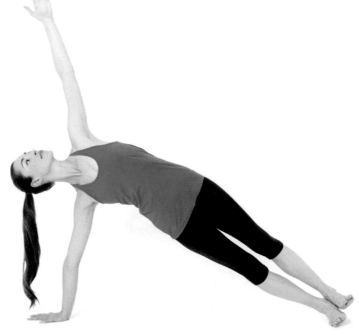

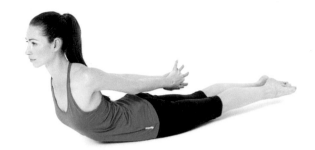

 ## INTERLACE HANDS BACK ARCH

From side plank, roll back to plank and ease your knees down to the ground. Bend your elbows and gently lower your body all the way to the ground. Interlace your hands behind you, palms together, take a big inhale, and lift your body off the ground. Extend the top of your head forward and keep the back of your neck nice and long. When you are ready, release your hands and gently lower down.

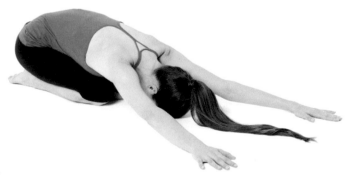

CHILD'S POSE

Press your palms into the ground and shift your hips back to sit on your heels. Extend your arms out in front of you and relax your forehead on the ground. Stay here for five deep breaths.

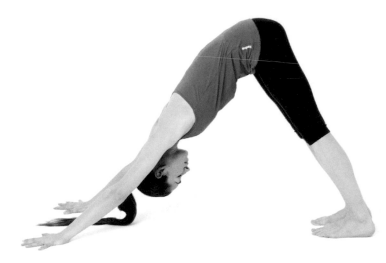

 ## DOWN DOG

Come onto all fours, tuck your toes, inhale, and lift your hips up and back to down dog. Relax your head, neck, and shoulders. Pedal through your feet and sway your body side to side, however feels great.

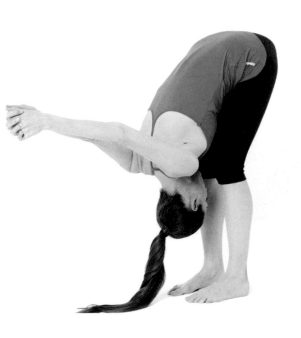

STANDING FORWARD BEND SHOULDER RELEASE

From down dog, slowly walk your feet up toward your hands. Don't worry about keeping your hands anchored in place—they can move, too, if that feels good. Step your feet parallel to each other a few inches apart and fold your torso over your legs. Bend your knees gently to release your lower back and hamstrings. Interlace your hands, palms together, behind you and relax your arms up and over your head. Take five long, deep breaths here.

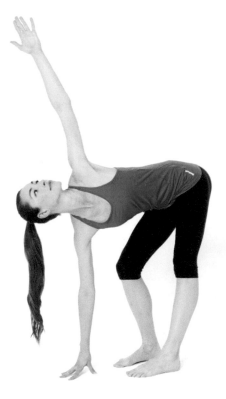

☆ STANDING FORWARD BEND BACK LENGTHENER

From standing forward bend, press your left fingertips on the ground a few inches in front of your feet. Soften both knees and open your body to your right side. Extend your right arm up above you and gaze up toward your right hand. Do the same on the other side.

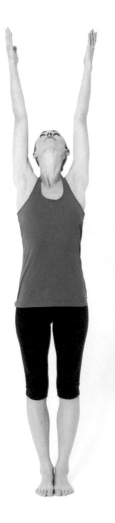

☆ STANDING ARM REACH

Roll up through your spine slowly, one vertebra at a time. When the top of your head lifts up, inhale as you open your arms out and up over your head.

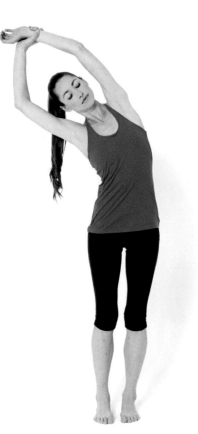

☆ STANDING EASY SIDE BEND

Grab your left wrist with your right hand. Inhale and lift your torso up so much that you arc over toward your right side, like a rainbow. Bend your knees slightly and allow your body to shift and drift, however it feels nice. Do the other side.

☆ STANDING FORWARD BEND WRIST RELEASE

Inhale, release your wrist, and lift both arms straight up. Exhale and roll down to a standing forward bend. Gently hang your torso over your legs. Bend your knees enough so you can step on your hands, so the tops of your hands are on the ground, toes up to your wrists. When you are ready, release your hands.

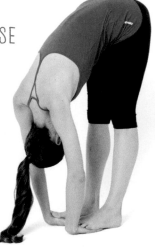

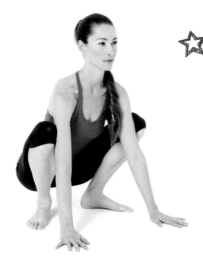

☆ SQUAT

Press your hands into the ground, point your toes out, and sink your heels and hips down into a squat. Either keep your hands on the ground for support or press the palms of your hands together to lengthen your back.

☆ SEATED BOTH LEGS FORWARD BEND

Press your hands behind your hips on the ground and ease yourself down to sit. Extend your legs out in front of you and soften your knees. Relax your torso over your legs. If you feel a struggle or tightness in your hamstrings, bend your knees even more so your torso is resting on your thighs. Relax your head and neck.

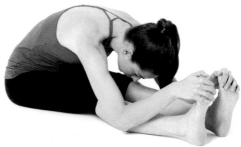

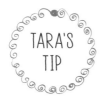

TARA'S TIP

DON'T OVERSTRETCH. FLEXIBILITY BEGINS IN THE MIND. ALLOW YOURSELF TO RELAX SO YOUR BODY CAN OPEN. IF YOU STRETCH FORCEFULLY, YOUR MIND TENSES UP AND SIGNALS YOUR BODY TO PROTECT AGAINST YOU, CREATING MORE TENSION. ALLOW YOUR MIND TO BE RELAXED AND YOUR BODY WILL OPEN WITH EASE.

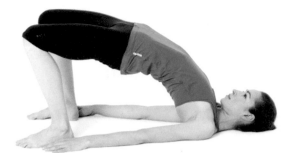

⭐ BRIDGE

Lie down on your back. Plant the bottoms of your feet on the ground next to your hips so your knees point up. Relax your arms down by your sides. Press into your arms and lift your hips up. Extend out through your chest and lengthen out through your knees. When you are ready, ease your body down one vertebra at a time.

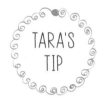

TARA'S TIP — NO ONE POSE IS BETTER THAN ANOTHER. A WHEEL IS NOT BETTER OR MORE ADVANCED THAN A BRIDGE. THE MOST IMPORTANT THING IS TO LISTEN TO YOUR BODY AND MOVE HOW YOU FEEL. THE GOAL IS TO CONNECT, NOT TO POSE.

⭐ WHEEL

From a resting position after bridge, if your back feels open and you'd like to come into wheel, press the palms of your hands on the ground outside your ears. Press down into your hands as you lift your hips and chest up. If you feel unsteady at all, gently relax down. If you feel steady, press through your arms and down through your feet to come into wheel. When you are ready to come down, tuck your chin lightly in toward your chest and gently roll down onto your back.

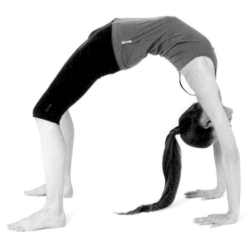

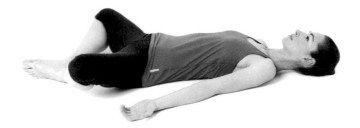

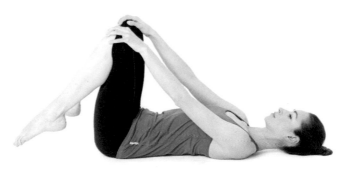

RECLINING BACK RELEASE

From a resting position after wheel or bridge, grab your knees with your hands. Allow your legs to fall away from your torso. You should feel a nice opening from the top of your head down through your tailbone.

RECLINING BOTH KNEES HUG

From reclining back release, hug your legs into your chest. Rock gently side to side to release your back.

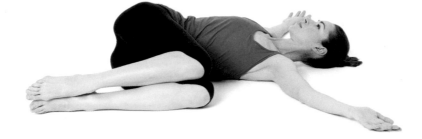

☆ RECLINING KNEES TOGETHER TWIST

From reclining both knees hug, gently lower both knees over toward your left side. Open your arms out to your sides. Gaze either upward or toward your right hand, however feels best on your back and neck. Then shift your knees and gaze to the opposite side.

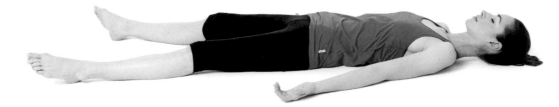

☆ RELAXATION

When you are ready, lie down to relax. Open your legs and arms a bit to your sides. Close your eyes. Take a big inhale through your nose. Exhale out through your mouth. Repeat this twice more. Return to normal breathing through your nose. Relax.

EASY SEATED

Start to bring a little more air back into your body. Move your fingers and toes around. Interlace your hands and take a nice stretch over your head. Hug your knees into your chest and rock up to sit up tall in easy seated position. Roll around a bit in your body until you find a nice, neutral balanced point. Close your eyes and take a few big deep breaths. When you are ready, open your eyes.

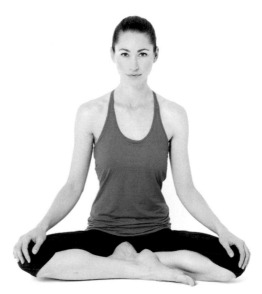

Great job! I hope you feel de-stressed, easy, open, and calm. I'm wishing you a restful evening of sweet dreams and a refreshed morning so you can start your day with all the energy and inspiration that is inside you naturally.

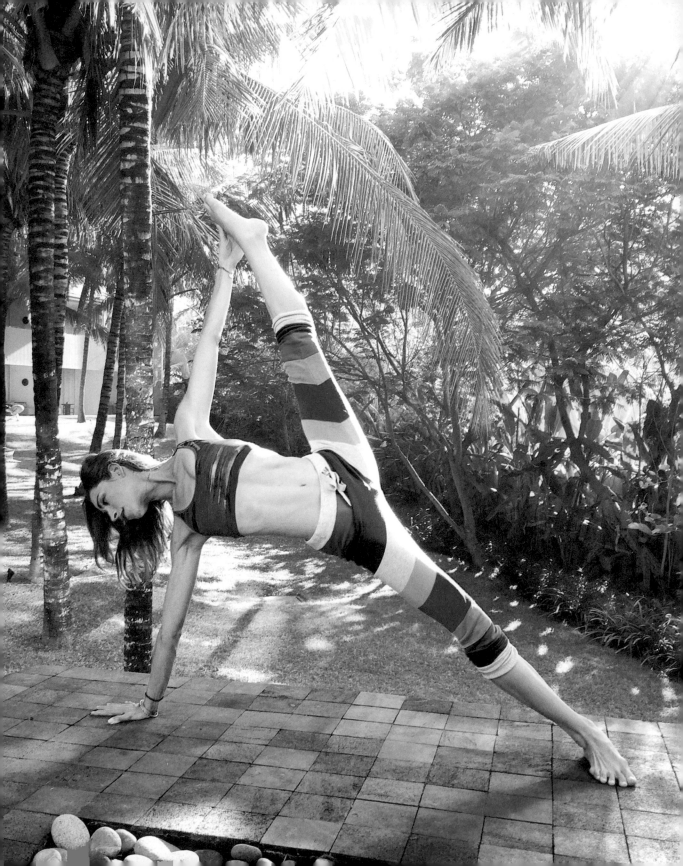

working your cushion

I've always been a physical person. I express myself with my hands and body enthusiastically when I speak. I love to move daily. Whether it's yoga, dancing, or walking around, I'm always moving. Having this physical outlet for my whole life is more about who I am than what I choose to do with my time. Movement has always been a meditation for me, and the way Strala is designed—to move easily with the breath during simple and challenging moments alike—shares that meditative experience with everyone who participates. Movement doesn't have to be separate from meditation. Your practice can be meditation. A walk in nature can be meditation. Gardening can be meditation. A ride on the subway can be meditation. Wherever we go and whatever we do is an opportunity to turn inward and reflect. And when we do this, space opens up and we feel calm, connected, and centered. From this centered place, we have new inspiration and energy to go out into the world and do what we do best. Meditation is a fantastic practice of awakening to ourselves. When we feel disconnected and off balance, a few moments of tuning in can open us up and ground us right back into that centered, inspired, happy place that we love. When we hold that happiness internally and stay connected, we can start to spill that joy into everything we do. Life becomes easy and light. It doesn't mean that challenges and hardships don't occur; it means we are more equipped to deal with everything that life presents us with more grace, compassion, and love. Who doesn't want that? I know, right? Good stuff.

While I do find meditation in my movement, I've also made a commitment to myself to do some sitting meditation each day, too. I actually sit on the ground (aka my two stacked Mexican blankets at home) and pay attention to my breath for a few moments. A good friend of mine, Mallika Chopra, who has been practicing meditation since she was a kid, taught by her dad, Deepak, reminds me every time I see her that I should meditate more. When I say that she reminds me, I don't mean that she tells me; rather, she inspires me by how calm and easy and open she is in her body, mind, and heart. By being around her and catching up on all of life, I am reminded that when I practice meditation regularly, I stay firmly rooted to my intention to connect and share with the world. Just like practicing yoga, the more you practice meditation, the better you feel from the inside out. So make a proper meditation date with yourself on a regular basis. It feels fantastic. I'm excited for you to fall in love with the process of meditation!

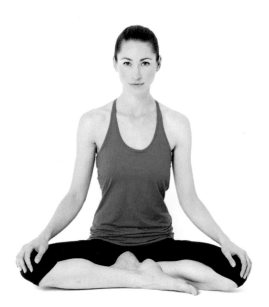

EASY BREATHING

Sit up tall, however you can sit comfortably. You don't have to be cross-legged like a picture in a yoga magazine. You can be on the couch, in a chair, or on the floor. However you are comfortable is great. Relax your hands on your thighs. Close your eyes, breathe in and out through your nose, and start to guide your attention inward. Deepen your inhales and lengthen your exhales. Set a nice, easy, full pace of breath that you can stay with for a while. Start to pay attention to your inhales and your exhales as they come and go. If you notice your mind wandering, guide your attention back to your breath. If you notice your mind wandering again, guide your attention back to your breath again. Continue breathing, watching, and guiding your attention back for five minutes. Keep a notebook handy for any deep thoughts. When you are finished, gently open your eyes.

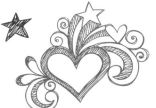

4 COUNT BREATHING

Counting the breath is a useful technique to give the mind something to do. If you find your mind wandering a lot with Easy Breathing, 4 Count Breathing, also called Box Breathing, might provide the bit of structure that does the trick. Sit up tall, however you can sit comfortably. Relax your hands on your thighs. Close your eyes and breathe in and out through your nose. Take a few big deep inhales and exhales to begin. Exhale all the air out. Take a long inhale as you count to four. Hold all the air at the top for another four count. Exhale all the air out for another four count. You can hold at the bottom also, if you wish. Some people don't like the feeling of keeping their lungs empty for four counts, but some like it quite a lot, so experiment to see what works for you. Continue breathing in this pattern for five minutes. When you are finished, gently open your eyes.

ALTERNATE NOSTRIL BREATHING

Alternate Nostril Breathing is a great way to put yourself and your nervous system at ease. It's nice to kick off a meditation session with a few rounds of Alternate Nostril Breathing and then transition to 4 Count or Easy Breathing. Of course, it's always totally up to you to try out different combinations and practice what works for you. Remember, you are different every day, so the same technique will feel different from day to day.

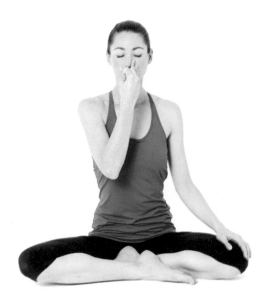

Sit up tall, however you can sit comfortably. Relax your hands on your thighs. Close your eyes and breathe in and out through your nose. Take a few big deep inhales and exhales to begin. On your right hand, curl the first two fingers (your peace fingers) into your palm so your ring finger, pinky, and thumb are pointing up. This leaves just enough space for your nose to fit in perfectly. Place your ring finger and pinky on the left side of your nose and the thumb on the right side. Close your right nostril with your thumb and take a big inhale through your left nostril. Close your left nostril with your ring finger, keeping your right side closed also, and hold all the air in for a few moments. Release your thumb (your right nostril) and let all the air out. Take a big inhale through your right side, close both sides, and hold closed for a few moments. Release the left side (ring finger side) and let all the air out. Continue to alternate between the sides. You can count the timing of the breath as in 4 Count Breathing if you like, or if you prefer to feel it out, that works, too. Continue to alternate for three to five minutes, then relax your hands back on your thighs. When you are finished, gently open your eyes.

HUG THE UNIVERSE—ARMS IN V

Meditating with your arms stretched in a V is an interesting practice that usually brings up quite a bit of physical sensation and the opportunity to choose how to deal with it. The neat thing about sitting with your arms in a V for a few minutes is that your arms will start to feel tired. You might have the desire to relax your arms, but you also know that nothing bad will happen if you keep them up. Your arms won't fall off, and it's just a few minutes of your time.

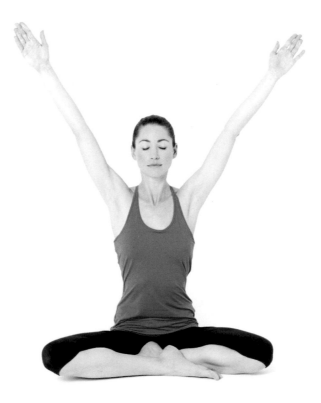

Sit up tall, however you can sit comfortably. Extend your arms up in a V. Close your eyes and pay attention to your breath. If you notice your mind wandering, guide your attention back to your breath. If you notice your arms beginning to tingle, guide your attention back to your breath. Continue for five minutes. When you are finished, slowly lower your hands onto your thighs, and gently open your eyes.

BREATH OF FIRE

Breath of Fire is a heat-building technique that gets your system going and is a nice way to kick-start you into feeling mode. It's also useful if you are cold and want to warm up your system. Good to know if you get stuck outside in the winter without a warm coat!

An easy way to describe this technique is rapid sniffing. Short and fast inhales and exhales through your nose. Let's give it a go. Sit up tall, however you can sit comfortably. Close your eyes and take a few big deep inhales and exhales through your nose to begin. When you are ready, begin short and fast inhales and exhales through your nose, pulling the air in and pushing it out. Continue for 30 seconds or a minute if you are comfortable. Work your way up to three to five minutes once you feel okay with the sensation. When you are finished, continue with Easy Breathing or 4 Count Breathing to round out your session for a few moments. Take note of any sensations as they come and go, guiding your attention back to your breath. When you are finished, gently open your eyes.

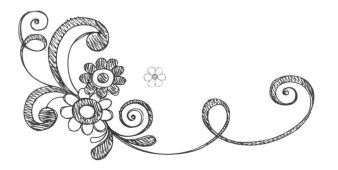

BELLOWS BREATHING

If Breath of Fire is like putting on a warm coat on a chilly day, Bellows Breathing is like building a giant bonfire on a warm summer's night. The sensation is hotter and has a deep cleansing effect. This technique involves forcefully pushing out your exhale and allowing your inhale to come on its own. It's like blowing your nose in a rapid repetition. You also might want to have a tissue handy if you have any sinus buildup. Bellows Breath is nice for clearing out the system. Let's try it.

Sit up tall, however you can sit comfortably. Close your eyes and take a few big deep inhales and exhales through your nose to begin. Take a big inhale, and begin short, fast exhales, allowing your inhales to come on their own. Either relax your hands on your thighs or place one hand on your lower belly to feel the pumping sensation of your belly moving in as you exhale and relaxing out as you inhale. Continue this breathing for 30 seconds to a minute if you are comfortable. Work your way up to three to five minutes once you feel okay with the sensation. When you are finished, continue with Easy Breathing or 4 Count Breathing to round out your session for a few moments. Take note of any sensations as they come and go, guiding your attention back to your breath. When you are finished, gently open your eyes.

MANTRA MEDITATIONS

Meditating with a mantra is another way to give your mind something to do while you pay attention to your breath. A mantra can be something simple, inspirational, and personal to you, or it can be a traditional mantra that has been used in meditations over the years. Most common are two-word mantras, one word recited on the inhale, and one word on the exhale. You can either say the word out loud or silently in your mind. Short phrases also work and don't need to be timed with the breath; they can be repeated gently, over and over.

Here are some simple mantras to try out. Feel free to make up your own.

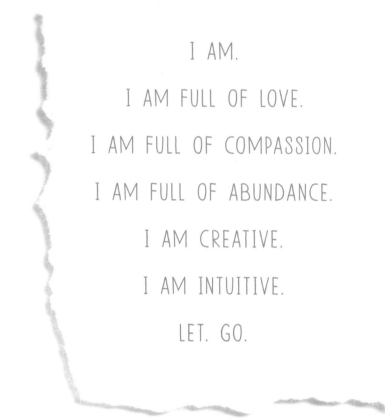

I AM.

I AM FULL OF LOVE.

I AM FULL OF COMPASSION.

I AM FULL OF ABUNDANCE.

I AM CREATIVE.

I AM INTUITIVE.

LET. GO.

Sit up tall, however you can sit comfortably. Close your eyes and take a few big deep inhales and exhales through your nose to begin. Start to softly speak your mantra of choice. If you feel uncomfortable saying it out loud, you can whisper it or say it in your mind. It's completely up to you. Continue to repeat your mantra while paying attention to your breath for three to five minutes and finish with a few moments of Easy Breathing. When you are finished, gently open your eyes.

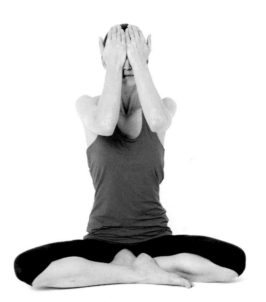

CALM EYES

A nice technique to calm your eyes and keep that nice meditation feeling going once you've opened your eyes is to put some warmth on your eyes and forehead. If you're like me, you'll fall in love with this technique and be doing it midday whenever you need a reset.

Rub the palms of your hands together quickly to get some heat going. Once you have some heat, close your eyes, press the heels of your hands gently on top of your eyes, and let your fingers rest on your forehead. Take a few big deep breaths here. When you are ready, relax your hands on your thighs and gently open your eyes.

KEEP EXPERIMENTING AND HAVE FUN

Whether you stick with some of these techniques or make up your own, keep experimenting to find what works for you, and know that it might change from day to day. Try keeping a meditation journal to keep track of your thoughts, ideas, and experiences. And, most important, remember to have fun. There might be moments that come easier than others, but allow yourself to enjoy the ride. Meditation is a practice for you to connect and feel into yourself. Stay on the path. You're on the right one!

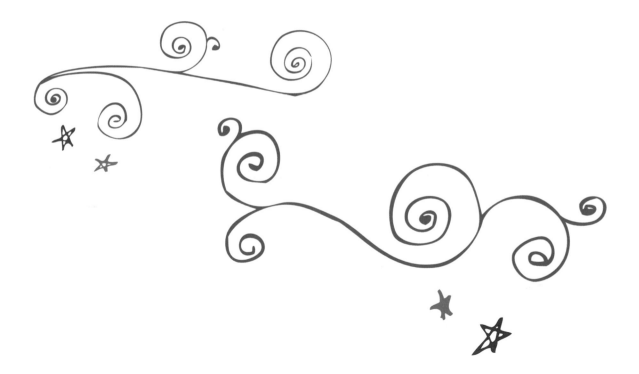

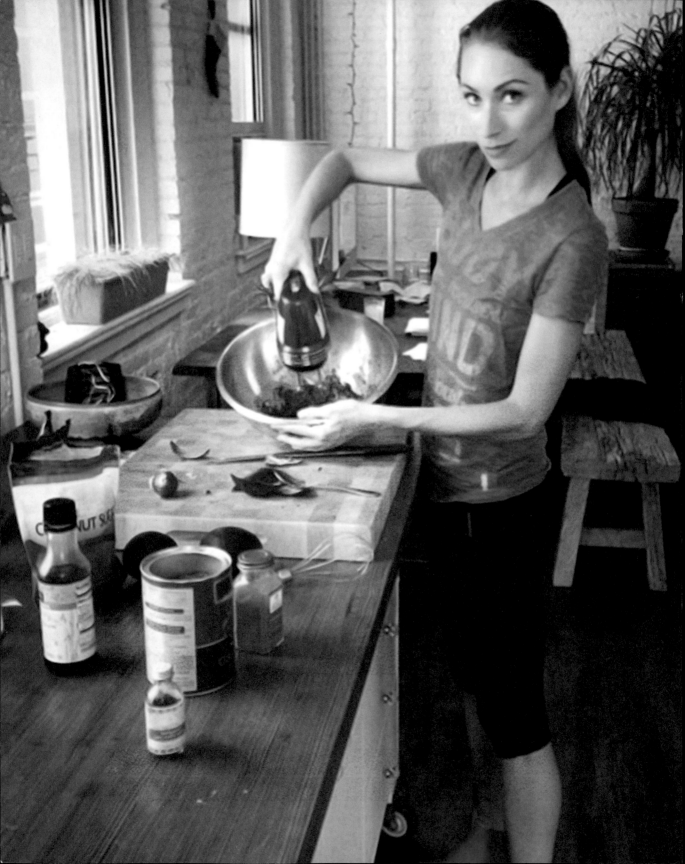

working
your kitchen

Have you worked up an appetite yet with all those yoga and meditation routines? Good! Now it's time to get in the kitchen and start whipping up some great-tasting food! The following drinks, snacks, meals, and treats are super-simple. I don't believe you need a huge list of ingredients and several hours to make something healthy and delicious. There are a lot of complicated recipes out there that might be impressive to pull off and enjoyable to eat, but I know for me,

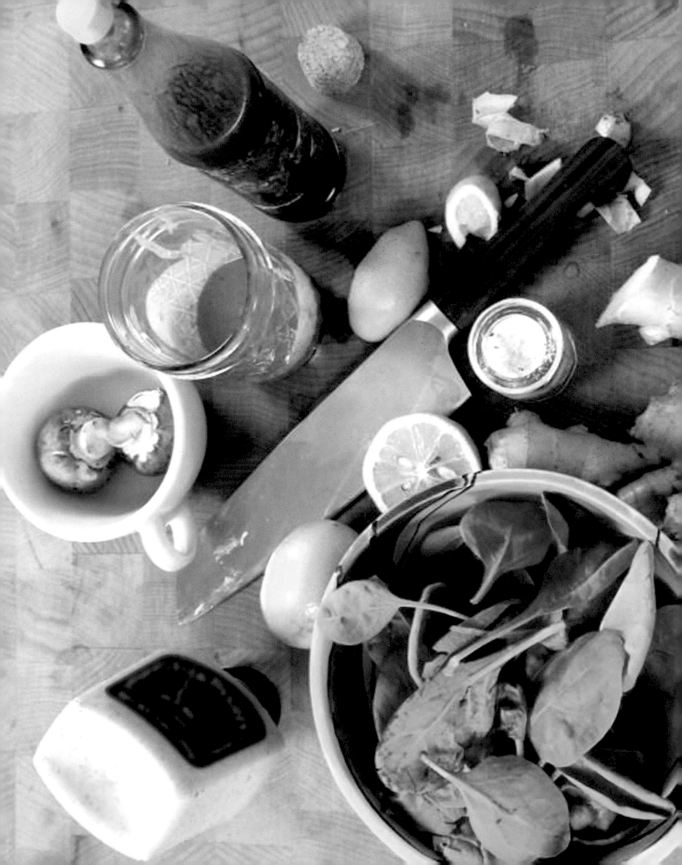

if there are simple ingredients, and if it's easy and relatively quick to prepare, I'm more likely to follow a recipe and make and enjoy it often. For the most part, when I look at a complicated, impressive recipe—filled with ingredients and kitchen gadgets that I don't already have—my journey ends with looking at the recipe. So here I present to you delicious, nutritious recipes that are straightforward. They've changed my life and opened me up to navigating the health food world in a doable way. Being radiant shouldn't have to be a hundred-step process filled with lots of rules. The beauty in health is finding your own rules and enjoying the elegance in simplicity.

Feeling great and living well can be quite easy when we allow ourselves the space to follow how we feel and make our own rules. I'll lay out some ideas, and you can modify them as you desire. Think of this like a coloring book—use your favorite colors and feel free to color outside the lines. The best artists always do! Add what you like, take out what you don't, and make your own rules. There is no one-size-fits-all diet. It's up to you to experiment and have a great time along the way.

Allow yourself the physical and mental space to be creative and enjoy the process. And allow your creativity to squish out in every direction. Daydream about comforting, relaxing breakfasts; energizing, satisfying lunches; and delicious, filling dinners that will leave you healthy and happy, and make your taste buds and tummy completely content and feeling fabulous. Just like in yoga, life, and everything else: stay easy and enjoy the ride!

So get your chef's hat on, and let's get our hands dirty and have some fun!

Time to eat!

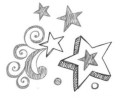

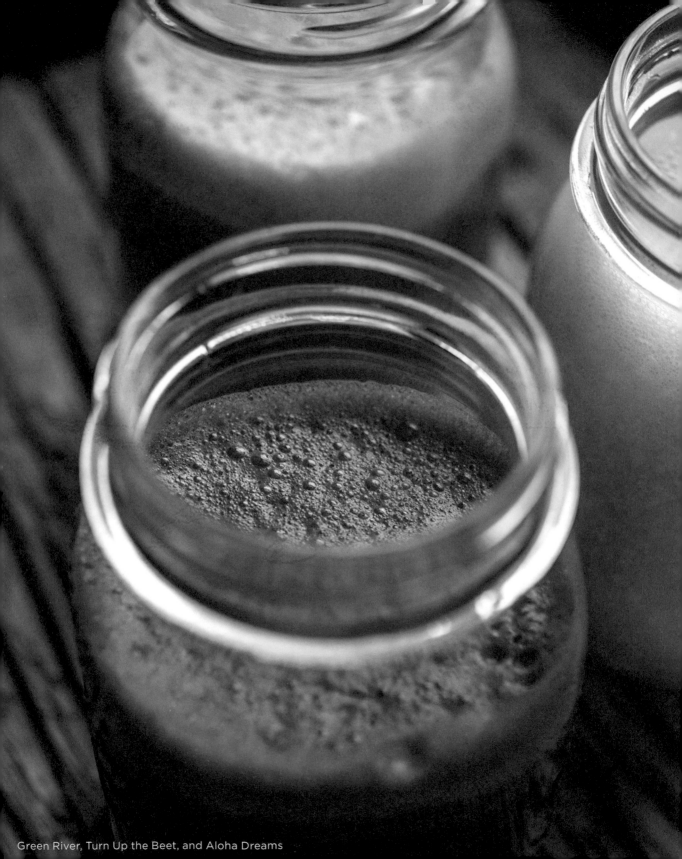

Green River, Turn Up the Beet, and Aloha Dreams

JUICE IT

Juice brands are everywhere, and the price per serving is high. Walking around my neighborhood in NYC, I pass by several juice shops in just a few blocks. Prices range from $6 to $15 per juice, give or take a few bucks. You can get a shiny new juicer of your own for the equivalent of eight or so store-bought juices, and then you can make hundreds of juices happily in the comfort of your own home.

Once I started making juice, I saw just how healthy it is. Because it's juice—not the whole vegetable—you can consume an awesomely healing amount of nutrients. Handfuls of greens and multiple fruits and vegetables go into each drink. Plus, since you've already extracted the nutrients from the vegetables, your body can easily absorb them. So, juice is like a crazy turbo shot of nutrients. It's like drinking sunshine. Plus, it'll make you glow like an angel. The secret for great skin, hair, nails, and eyes that sparkle doesn't come in cream form from the beauty supply store; it's in your mug o' greens.

With juicing you'll get other benefits, too, such as improved sleep, weight loss and management, healthy digestion, improved mood, improved immunity, bright eyes, glowing skin, healthy hair, improved clarity, and general happiness. I'm letting you know from experience that all these benefits are very real. I went from drinking Mountain Dew for energy to swapping it out with juices. It's not the caffeine that gives you sustained energy. It's the plants!

When I started experimenting with making juices, I just mixed greens and added in some other fruits and veggies for nutritional value and volume. I found that apples have this amazing quality of making a juice frothy, like a cappuccino. Celery and cucumber are great ways to "fill out" a green juice. Plus, cucumber adds a nice smooth tone. Or, you could throw in some ginger for a spicy kick! Just remember, it's all about figuring out what you like—so play around. Have fun. Make your own juice rules.

GREEN RIVER

When I was a kid, we would sometimes go on vacations up in Chicago, aka the big city. We'd see a baseball game or just wander around and check out all the tall buildings. On these trips, we often went to Ed Debevic's, a superfun 1950s-themed restaurant. There was always so much action in that place. The waitresses rode on roller skates and wore pink-striped jumpsuits. There was a jukebox blasting oldies, and 1950s nostalgia covered every inch of the restaurant. Everything about it was like a theatrical production, and I thought it was magical.

Every time I went there, I would order a drink called Green River, named that because the Chicago River was dyed green. It came in a huge glass that was bigger than my head. Who knows what was in it? Probably just a mixture of Sprite and green food coloring. What I do know—100 percent for sure—was that it was not healthy.

Since the best part of the experience for me was saying, "I'd like a Green River, please," I figured I could keep that part. So here, my friends, is an updated, überhealthy Green River for you. Kale is packed with vitamins A, C, and K, so it's chock-full of goodness and it tastes great, too. For all of you out there that believe green juice is nasty, bland stuff, I hope this concoction will revolutionize your perspective. Have a Green River, please!

SERVES 2

2 big handfuls kale with the stems, broken into manageable pieces
½ cucumber, chopped
1 apple, any variety, chopped
½-inch ginger, peeled
½ lemon, sliced in half

Juice everything except the lemon.
Squeeze lemon on top of the juice.

ENJOY!

TURN UP THE BEET

On my journey down the rabbit hole of taking care of myself—going inside and paying attention to how I feel—I started thinking about all the stuff we are made of, and I kept coming back to blood. We've got several quarts of the stuff flowing through us like a river. I know vitamins in plants are great for keeping our bodies and minds strong and clear, but what about our blood? In asking around, the answer kept coming back to beets. Finally, I got up the courage to put a few of those bad boys in my shopping cart and give it a go. What I discovered was my absolute favorite color—the most vibrant, beautiful hot pink ever. I loved the color and texture, and rings like those of an old wise tree were an added bonus.

SERVES 2

1 beet, chopped
3 carrots, chopped
½-inch ginger, peeled and sliced

Juice all ingredients.

ENJOY!

THE POPEYE

Spinach has been one of my all-time favorite foods since I was a little kid. At the mall in my hometown, there were these rotating salad bars where we often ate. I would walk around the wheel of food in buckets—instead of standing still and waiting for food to come to me—because I was in search of one thing only: spinach! Well, to be honest, I was looking for chocolate pudding, too, but spinach came first. I had a lot I wanted to do, and I knew spinach would help me get there—just like it helped Popeye. Also, I loved the taste and how it made me feel.

Lucky for me, spinach is at the top of nutrient richness. Boasting loads of vitamins K, A, C, B1, and B3, plus calcium, potassium, iron, copper, and zinc, it's like a whole lot of science project awesomeness in these gorgeous green leaves. Spinach also contains glycoglycerolipids, which have anti-inflammatory properties that help protect our bodies from things like digestive tract issues, bone problems, and even cancers. Strong to the finish!

I hope you get hooked on this juice as much as I am and we can become like Popeye together!

SERVES 2

4 handfuls spinach
½ apple, any variety, chopped
½ cucumber, chopped
2 stalks celery
½-inch ginger, sliced and peeled

Juice all ingredients.

ENJOY!

ALOHA DREAMS

Pineapples are such a happy-looking fruit. With the wild hair spiking out the top and the fun, groovy shape, they look like a party. Juicing a pineapple is a sweet treat, so I do this rarely—mostly when someone visits my home on a hot summer day. This makes even more sense when you think about the fact that the pineapple has been a symbol of welcome for many centuries all over the world.

If you have an organic pineapple, it's fun to juice the skin, as well. This adds a frothy cappuccino-like topping. I like to serve this juice over ice and toss a few thin slices of strawberries on top for extra presentation points. Sometimes I go crazy and just throw some strawberries in the juicer for some extra color.

SERVES 4

1 pineapple, cored and chopped
Juice of 3 limes
4 strawberries, sliced with the tops removed

Juice the whole pineapple.
Add lime juice and a handful of ice.
Stir.
Top with strawberries.

ENJOY!

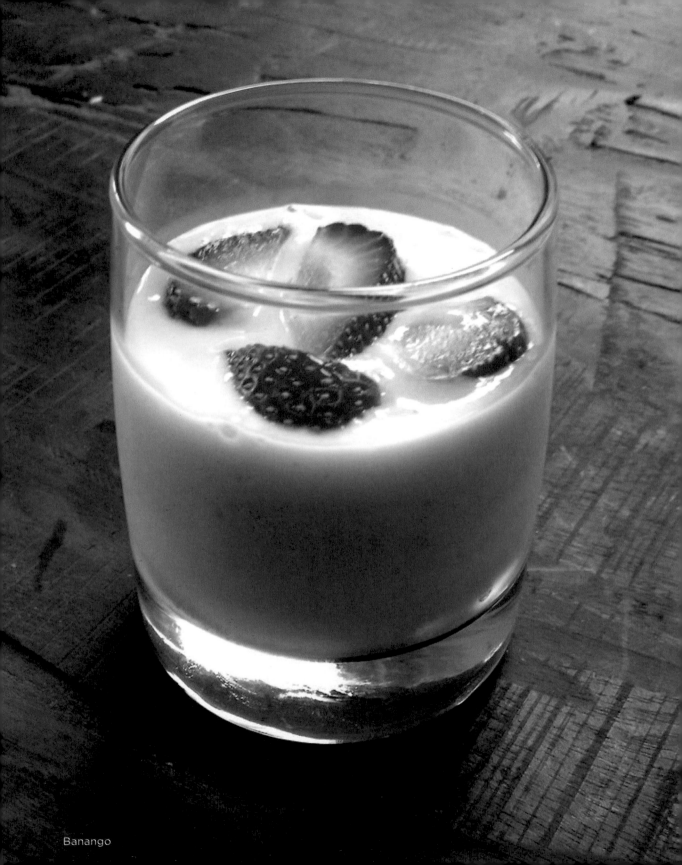

Banango

BLEND IT

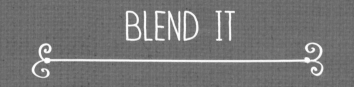

A smoothie off the street will set you back in the same ballpark as a juice. DIY at home is for sure a great way to go. Just like with juice, you can experiment, learn, and create your own magical creations. It's fun and empowering to make edible healing creations yourself.

One great thing about having a smoothie instead of juice is that you keep the fiber. I like to alternate between drinking juices and smoothies because sometimes I need that turbo shot of nutrients and sometimes I want a more filling "meal in a glass" that sustains me a bit longer. Before I lead or take a class at the studio, most days I choose a smoothie, because I need the extra something-something I get from keeping all the ingredients in the glass. When I don't have to be as physical or after a yoga class, it's nice to drink a juice. You'll find your own rhythm of what works great for you.

And just like juice, smoothies give you those added benefits regarding sleep, immunity, skin, energy, and so on. I'm excited for your blending adventures!

CLEMENTINE CREAMSICLE

Growing up I drank a big glass of milk with every meal and ate a big bowl of ice cream every night for dessert. Dairy was front and center for every meal and every treat, and I loved every bit of it. Knowing what we know now about dairy, my childhood seems like a completely different era. So much has changed. But that doesn't mean I've stopped loving those delicious creamy desserts. Ice cream is still a favorite treat of mine—but most of the time, I try to find a different (healthier) way to satisfy those cravings.

This Clementine Creamsicle reminds me of the gallon of multicolored sherbet my family kept stocked in the Deepfreeze in our basement. But now I can enjoy it without the tummyache.

SERVES 2

1 frozen banana* or 1 nonfrozen banana and 6 ice cubes
4 clementines or 1 orange, peeled
½ cup almond milk

Blend it.

ENJOY!

*Make sure to peel the banana before you freeze it!

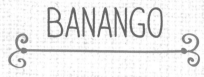

BANANGO

Bananas are a lifesaver for me. Whether I grab one on the go or blend one up in a tasty, nutritious drink, bananas have staying power to keep me energized and focused no matter what the day brings. They have tons of potassium, which protects your cardiovascular system. Plus bananas can stop those insane muscle cramps that can come from not having enough potassium. Aside from the health benefits, I've found that coupling bananas with other exciting and yummy fruits delivers a blended snack that rivals some of the best desserts. One of my favorite pairings is mango. I dare you not to get hooked on the Banango!

SERVES 2

1 frozen banana* or 1 nonfrozen banana and 6 ice cubes
1 cup frozen mango
½ cup almond milk
2 strawberries, sliced (optional)

Blend it, then transfer to glasses and top with strawberries.

ENJOY!

*Make sure to peel the banana before you freeze it!

HEALTHY FROSTY

My hometown is like many that are built off a highway exit. When you enter, you are greeted by every major fast-food chain known to America, a few family-owned restaurants, and a few gas stations. For the most part, my family didn't eat fast food. But occasionally we would indulge in a Wendy's Frosty, and man they were good! While I was changing my life—focusing on getting healthy—I accidently blended something together that tasted suspiciously similar to the Frosty. So I made it my mission to make it taste even more like one. I kept experimenting until I mastered it. Whether you miss and crave a Frosty or not, this healthy treat is so indulgent you won't have to look any further.

SERVES 2

1 frozen banana* or 1 nonfrozen banana and 6 ice cubes
1 cup almond milk
2 heaping tablespoons almond butter
1 tablespoon cocoa powder
1 teaspoon vanilla extract
1 teaspoon cinnamon
1 tablespoon maple syrup

Blend it.

ENJOY!

*Make sure to peel the banana before you freeze it!

THIN MINTS GIRL SCOUT SMOOTHIE

It's not a big argument about which Girl Scout cookies are the best. Thin Mints cookies totally rule the cookie drive—and the hearts of millions. The sales go to a good cause, but the consumption of entire boxes at a time does a number on our health. And let's be honest, it's impossible to eat just one . . . or just five! Mint chocolate is one of my favorite combinations on the planet, and this smoothie is amazing. I hope you love it as much as I do.

SERVES 2

1 frozen banana* or 1 nonfrozen banana and 6 ice cubes
1 cup almond milk
1 ounce dark chocolate**
6 ice cubes
1 teaspoon peppermint extract

Blend it.

ENJOY!

*Make sure to peel the banana before you freeze it!

**If you want to get really crazy, you can toss in a couple cookies instead of dark chocolate.

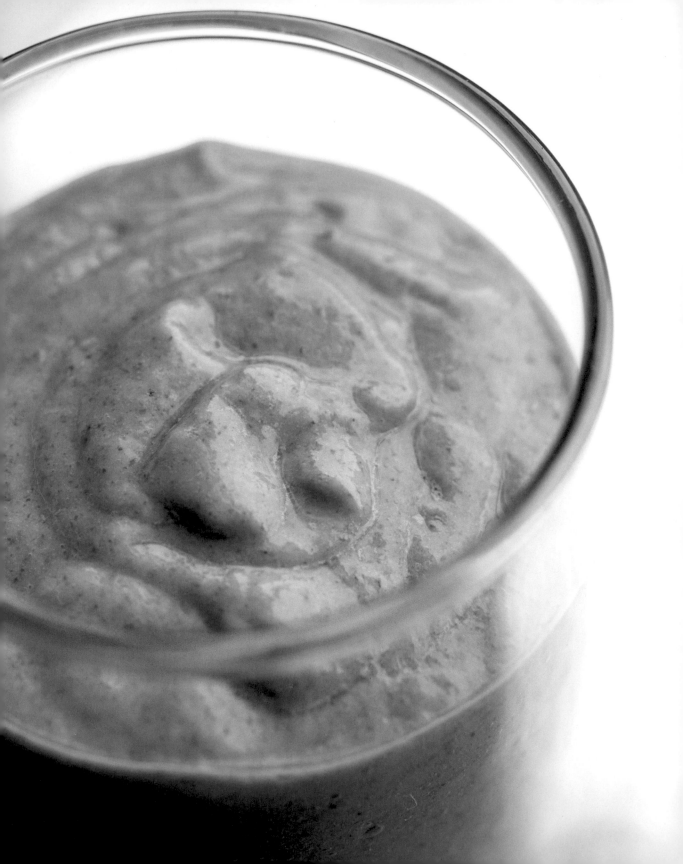

THE SWAMP

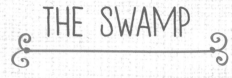

When you don't have time to sit down at the table and enjoy a balanced meal, you can whip one up and take it in your to-go mug. The Swamp has been a savior of mine on so many occasions when I haven't had enough time to prepare a proper meal. This smoothie includes all the vitamins and minerals of the greens, plus the potassium of the banana and the healthy fat of an avocado. It really is like a full meal, and while I don't recommend replacing all your meals with smoothies, this is a great way to get in the good stuff—instead of grabbing something unhealthy—when you are on the go.

SERVES 2

1 handful spinach
1 handful kale with stems, broken up into manageable pieces
1 frozen banana* or 1 nonfrozen banana and 6 ice cubes
1 avocado
2 cups almond milk

Blend it.

ENJOY!

*Make sure to peel the banana before you freeze it!

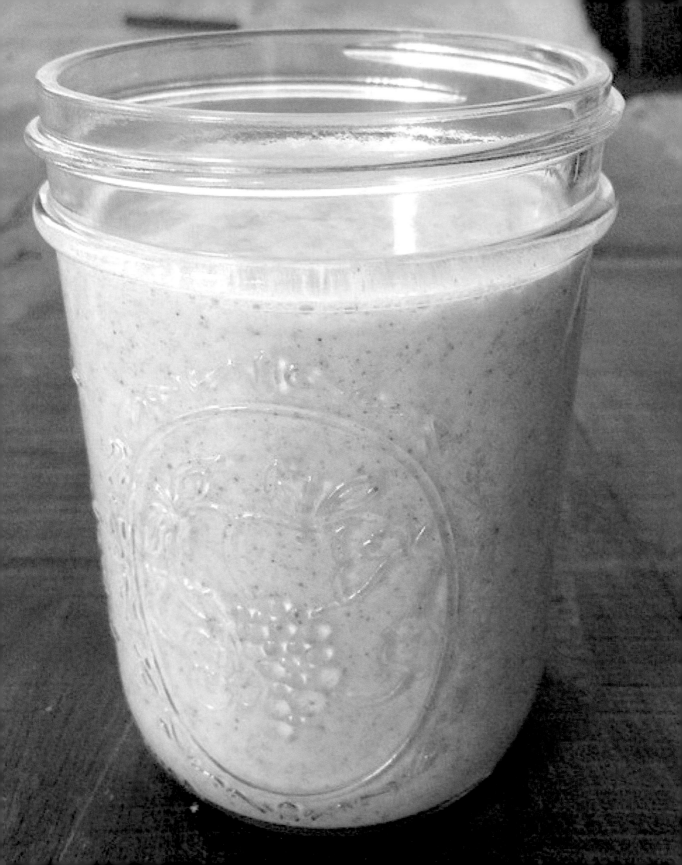

CHOCOLATE ALMOND BUTTER PROTEIN BOMB

If chocolate and peanut butter are as yummy together for you as they are for me, you're going to adore this ridiculously decadent, healthy treat. Eating healthy doesn't have to be bland, boring, and miserable. Once I cut all the junk out of my diet and started playing around with great ingredients, I realized that eating healthy actually tastes better than the junk food—and this is one of the drinks that made that oh-so-obvious for me. Plus, healthy food leaves you feeling energized for the short term, and radiantly healthy for the long term. All around, it's better. When you combine great ingredients like almond butter and chocolate, and toss in a few simple and healthy accessories, you win it all: taste, energy, and lasting health. Cheers to you!

SERVES 2

- 1 frozen banana* or 1 nonfrozen banana and 6 ice cubes
- 1 cup almond milk
- 1 heaping tablespoon almond butter
- 1 tablespoon cocoa powder
- 1 tablespoon plant-based protein powder (optional)

Blend it.

ENJOY!

*Make sure to peel the banana before you freeze it!

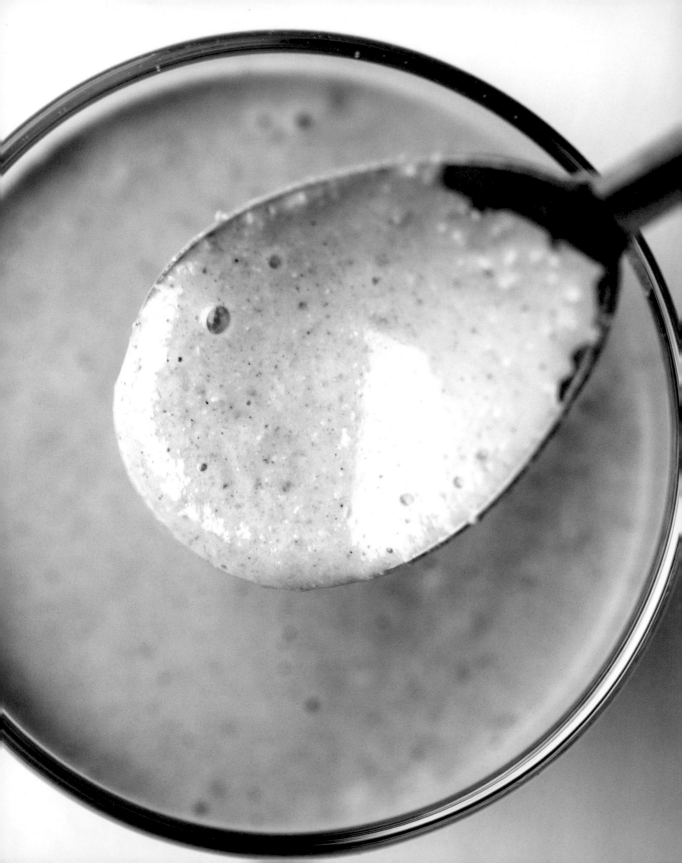

STRAWBERRY SHORTCAKE SMOOTHIE

I was more into playing outside than playing with dolls when I was young, but presents from family members usually came in the form of Barbies, Cabbage Patch Kids, Care Bears, Holly Hobbie, Raggedy Ann, and Strawberry Shortcake. I faked an interest to avoid appearing ungrateful to my generous relatives, but in all honesty, dolls just weren't my thing. However, I do have a soft spot for Strawberry Shortcake—mostly because she consistently smelled so yummy and fruity. On a visit home years after I got her, I found her in a closet and she still carried her sweet fruit smell.

My soft spot for Strawberry Shortcake, the doll, also applies to strawberry shortcake, the food. My mom makes a "healthy" version of this dessert, which is basically angel food cake with strawberries on top. As a child, I loved it. It smelled and tasted delicious. I still eat it up whenever it's around; however, when I'm not able to visit home, I have an even healthier version to satisfy me—and this one comes in a glass.

SERVES 2

1½ cups frozen strawberries or 1 cup nonfrozen strawberries and 1 cup ice
1 cup rolled oats
1 cup cashews
1 cup almond milk
1 tablespoon maple syrup
1 teaspoon vanilla extract
1 teaspoon cinnamon

Blend it.

ENJOY!

CREAMY EGGLESS NOG

My grandma and all my uncles and aunts live on one road in southern Illinois, and when we have a holiday, we usually visit everyone by going from house to house. One stop on this route is the home of Marge and Leon—even though they're not relatives, just good family friends. I remember one time as a kid scooting up to their kitchen table, grabbing a glass of creamy yellow liquid, and being told that it was eggnog and that it was good. To me it just smelled like eggs in a glass. I thought it was some sort of cruel joke. I took a tiny sip and was utterly grossed out—in the overly dramatic way that only six-year-olds are grossed out. I convulsed and made faces and vowed never to touch the stuff again. Well, of course, I grew out of that phase, and somewhere along the line I tried eggnog again, and the experience was much more pleasurable. But eggnog isn't known to be the healthiest drink on the planet, so I decided to create a version that's a lot lighter on the tummy. Plus . . . no raw eggs!

SERVES 2

1 cup almond milk
1 frozen banana* or 1 nonfrozen banana and 6 ice cubes
½ cup cashews
1 tablespoon maple syrup
1 teaspoon nutmeg
1 teaspoon cinnamon
1 teaspoon vanilla

Blend it.

ENJOY!

*Make sure to peel the banana before you freeze it!

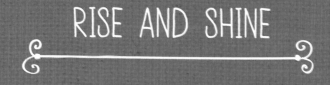

RISE AND SHINE

I'll be honest with you, even though breakfast is the most important meal of the day, I'm often guilty of skipping it when I have an early and busy morning. I'll at least try to squeeze in a smoothie or a juice, but sometimes the snooze button wins over a healthy, hearty morning meal. On the days when I rise and shine naturally after a full night's sleep, I make sure to prioritize one of these nutritious breakfasts to sustain my energy levels and keep me happy all morning long.

And the beauty of breakfast—for me—is that it always reminds me of my dad—especially if I have it for dinner. When I was a kid, if my mom wasn't around to make dinner—which rarely happened; we were spoiled—my dad was on dinner duty. And his favorite meal, I'm still convinced, is breakfast, because that's what he always made. Looking back, the toast and eggs he cooked up for my brother and me were probably a lot simpler than putting something in the pressure cooker for an hour. So even if I miss out on some goodness in the morning, I sometimes take a page out of my dad's playbook. He made his own breakfast rules, and now I make mine. And you can, too; so enjoy your rise and shine anytime!

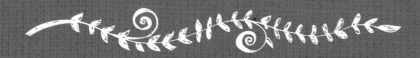

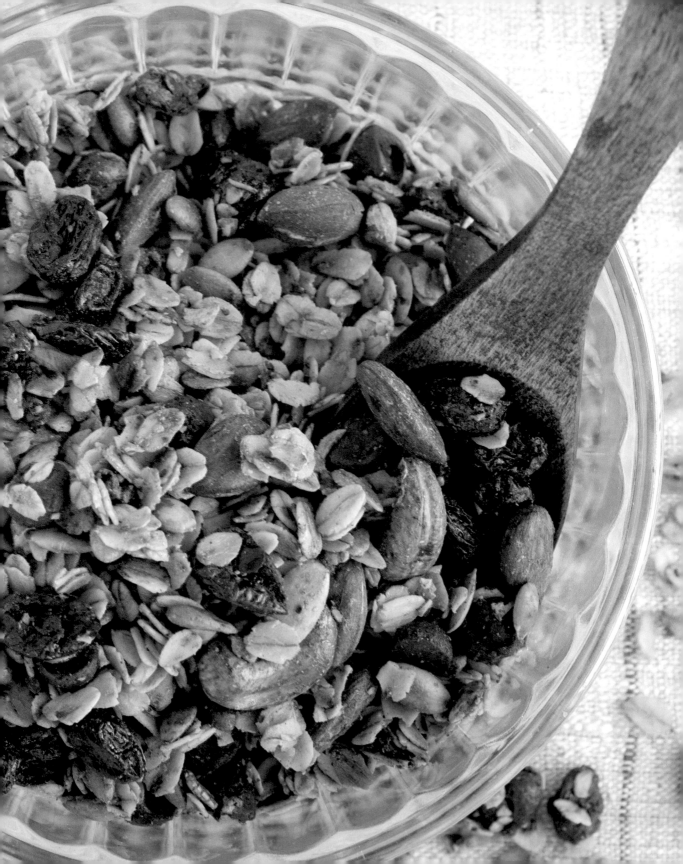

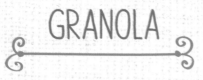

GRANOLA

I think it's common when first moving out on your own to go on a boxed and canned diet of cereal and soup. It's quick and easy to make, and, while it's not great for you, it cures hunger and gives you just enough energy to do what you need to do. Personally, I ran on Frosted Mini-Wheats for a few years. I suppose it gave me some essential calories and a few vitamins, but I know I could have felt better, and I probably could have been a lot more efficient in my life if I'd cooked and prepared food at home. This homemade granola, like store-bought cereal, is easy to keep on hand for those days when you're short on time. Plus, it's a crowd pleaser. I love to make a big batch, eat some, store some for later, and pack a few jars as gifts for friends. Feeding friends and family is a great reward, especially when they keep asking for more!

SERVES 10

4 cups rolled oats
½ cup sour cherries
1 cup mixture of almonds, dark chocolate chips, cashews, and sunflower seeds
½ cup coconut oil
½ cup maple syrup
1 tablespoon cinnamon

Preheat oven to 350 degrees Fahrenheit.
Mix all the ingredients well, making sure the oil and syrup are evenly distributed
    throughout the mixture.
Spread the mixture out on cookie sheet.
Bake for 25 minutes.
Let the granola cool completely.
Store the leftovers in covered glass containers.

ENJOY!

HOT FRUIT BOWL

Warm fruit for breakfast is as comforting as pie, and it's an energizing wholesome meal. It's filled with vitamins and antioxidants to get your day started right. The combination of fruits in this recipe is my favorite, but it's also easy to mix and match whatever fruit you have on hand. This dish is especially good in the winter months because it creates some extra warm fuzzies in the tummy. It's great served all by itself or topped with granola. You can also couple it with French toast if you're looking to make an impressive spread for guests—or for yourself. You're worth it, after all.

SERVES 2

5 strawberries, chopped
¼ cup blueberries
1 Gala apple, chopped
1 banana, chopped
1 teaspoon cinnamon

Combine all the fruits into a medium saucepan.
Cook over medium heat, stirring constantly for 5 minutes.
Remove from heat, transfer to serving bowls, and top with cinnamon.

ENJOY!

SPICY AVOCADO TOAST

When I was a kid, I would have thought avocado on toast would be the strangest thing to eat, especially for breakfast. Now that I'm all grown up, savory breakfasts are some of my favorite foods in the world. Spicing up the average avocado toast with jalapeño, hot sauce, and a few other special ingredients has evolved from a simple treat into my go-to when I know I have a big day ahead. It's a major energy booster, and it gives me the fuel that my body and mind need to get through the day. Plus, the spicy kick is a superfun way to wake up. It also reminds me that you really can make your own rules—have hot sauce for breakfast if you want!

SERVES 2

2 slices bread*
1½ teaspoons nondairy buttery spread
1½ teaspoons tomato paste
1 avocado
¼ jalapeño pepper, chopped
4 shakes hot sauce
1 teaspoon red pepper flakes
1 pinch sea salt
Juice of ½ lime

Toast the bread.
Spread nondairy buttery spread and tomato paste on the toast.
Mash the avocado with a fork in a small bowl.
Spread the avocado on the toast, and top with the jalapeño, hot sauce,
   red pepper flakes, sea salt, and lime juice.

ENJOY!

* You can use any type of bread for this recipe, but my favorite is Ezekiel bread.
It's made with sprouted grains, which means that your body can digest it more easily.

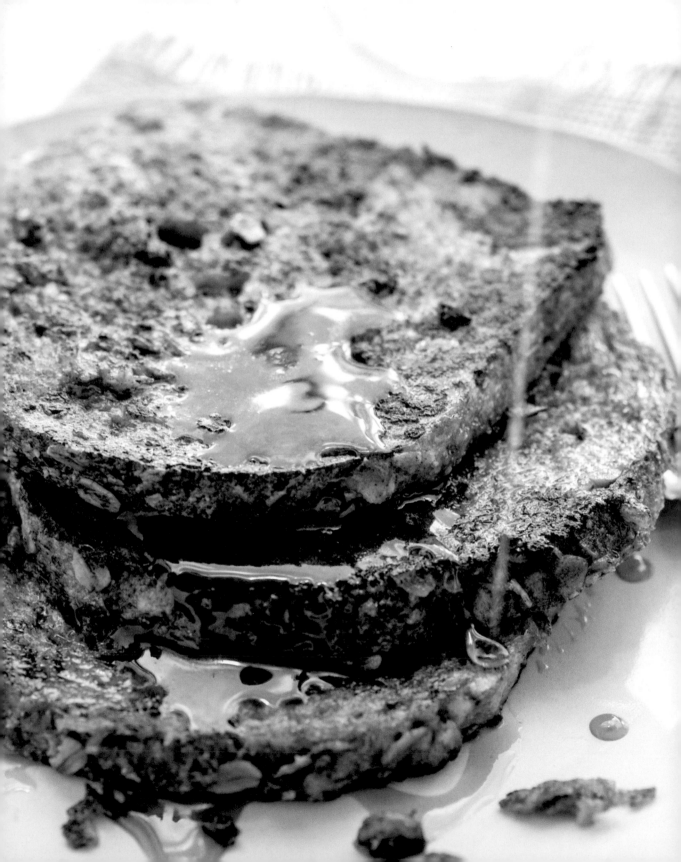

MAPLE FRENCH TOAST

A lazy weekend morning is something I fantasize about. With my busy life, I usually end up grabbing a breakfast smoothie on the go and jetting to the studio, but when I have time, I savor it. Reading the paper or a good book and cooking up some French toast with all the fixin's is my ideal lazy morning. And this French toast recipe is one of my all-time favorites. It not only tastes amazing but also is superhealthy. I hope you enjoy my favorite morning treat.

SERVES 2

2 bananas
1 cup almond milk
1 tablespoon nondairy buttery spread
4 to 5 slices bread*
1 tablespoon cinnamon, plus more for topping
4 tablespoons maple syrup

Combine the bananas and almond milk in a bowl by mashing them together with a fork or using a hand mixer set on low.

Heat a cast-iron skillet on medium heat.

Add the nondairy buttery spread to the skillet.

Dip the bread in banana mixture, and place it on the skillet.

Sprinkle cinnamon on top of bread while it cooks.

Flip the bread after it has browned, about 2 minutes.

Sprinkle cinnamon on the other side.

Remove the toast from skillet after it has browned on the other side, about 2 minutes.

Top with cinnamon and maple syrup.

ENJOY!

* You can use any type of bread for this recipe, but my favorite is Ezekiel bread. It's made with sprouted grains, which means that your body can digest it more easily.

SNACK ON IT

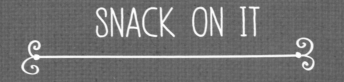

Snacks have always been an important part of my life. When I was a kid my mom would pick me up after school and drop me off for a good chunk of the afternoon and evening at dance class. She was always so nice to bring me a healthy snack of green peppers and carrots from the garden, or some nuts and maybe a homemade cookie for a treat. I'd usually be at dance until after dinnertime. Either Mom or Dad would be on duty to come and pick me up and as soon as I walked in they would reheat a plate of leftovers for me. Ah, the good life.

Grown-up life isn't so different, except now I'm in charge of feeding myself. My days are often filled, from class at the studio to the airport to an event or a meeting, and I wouldn't survive without healthy fuel on hand. When I have time at home, fixing snacks is just as fun as preparing whole meals. I eat when I'm hungry, and don't worry about if it's necessarily lunch or dinnertime. Part of being so physically active and having a practice of building intuition and awareness from the inside out is being able to listen to your body and know what it needs to feel nurtured. The following are a few of my favorite wholesome and delicious snacks that you can make when you just need a little something hearty and satisfying to carry you through your day.

SPINACH CASHEW MIX

Sometimes it's not time to eat, but *it's time to eat,* if you know what I mean. Sometimes you just can't wait until your next big meal, so you have to improvise. This happens to me a lot when I'm at home working on a project, often staring at my computer screen for way too long. I like to get up, take breaks, do a few down dogs, and make a healthy snack to keep me energized and clear. I came up with this yummy combo one day when the kitchen was pretty bare but I still had some spinach and cashews. I love this accidental snack because of how quick it is to make, how great it tastes, and also how jazzed up it makes me feel.

SERVES 1

1½ teaspoons nondairy buttery spread
2 big handfuls spinach
1 teaspoon red pepper flakes, or to taste
1 pinch sea salt
½ cup of cashews

Melt the nondairy buttery spread over medium heat in a cast-iron skillet.
Toss in the spinach and stir until it's wilted.
Mix in cashews and stir constantly for 1 minute.
Transfer the spinach to a serving bowl and toss with red pepper flakes and sea salt.

ENJOY!

SAVORY & SPICY MUSHROOM BITES

I often find myself hungry, wandering in the kitchen, down to only a few scraps of food, and wondering what I can pull off with what I have left. I came up with this fun combo on a creative whim, half inspired by the small mystery snacks I see passed around at events and half inspired by throwing a little party for myself at home. To create these tasty bites of goodness, I sliced up what I had and started assembling whatever I could. Because my Midwest influence hasn't left me entirely, I have the instinct to pile things in sandwich-like structures. I hope you enjoy these healthy, savory snacks. I often serve them up when friends come over and they always go fast; that's a good sign.

SERVES 2

1 handful spinach, chopped
½ tablespoon balsamic vinegar
¾ teaspoon extra-virgin olive oil
2 shakes hot sauce
3 tablespoons hummus
4 cremini mushrooms, sliced horizontally
¼ red bell pepper, sliced

Mix the spinach with the balsamic vinegar, olive oil, and hot sauce.
Spread the hummus on the mushroom slices.
Add a few spinach leaves to half of the mushroom slices.
Top with the bell pepper slices.
Place the mushroom caps on top to form sandwiches.

ENJOY!

FRESH GUACAMOLE

Like most people I know, I have a serious soft spot for Mexican food. The food reflects the culture—it's so fun, spicy, and full of life. Enjoying some fresh guacamole and a plate of rice and beans always makes me feel as if I'm part of the celebration. But Mexican food can be known to cause bellyaches—especially if you wash it down with pitchers of margaritas. Even though my healthy lifestyle has shifted toward fewer bellyaches and hangovers, I'm still hooked on guacamole. This recipe is a bit different from your standard guac. I discovered it one day when I had some leftover olives. I decided to toss those in and, even more surprising, the leftover olive juice at the bottom of the jar. This little alteration added so much flavor that I had to share it!

SERVES 2

1 avocado
¼ red onion, chopped
1 jalapeño, chopped
6 olives, chopped
1 tablespoon olive juice
Juice of ½ lemon
Juice of 1 lime
Blue tortilla or flax chips, or 2 cups chopped veggies

Mash the avocado with a fork in a small bowl, and stir in the onion, jalapeño, olives, and olive juice.

Toss in the lemon and lime juices and mash them in with a fork.

Serve with chips or veggies.

ENJOY!

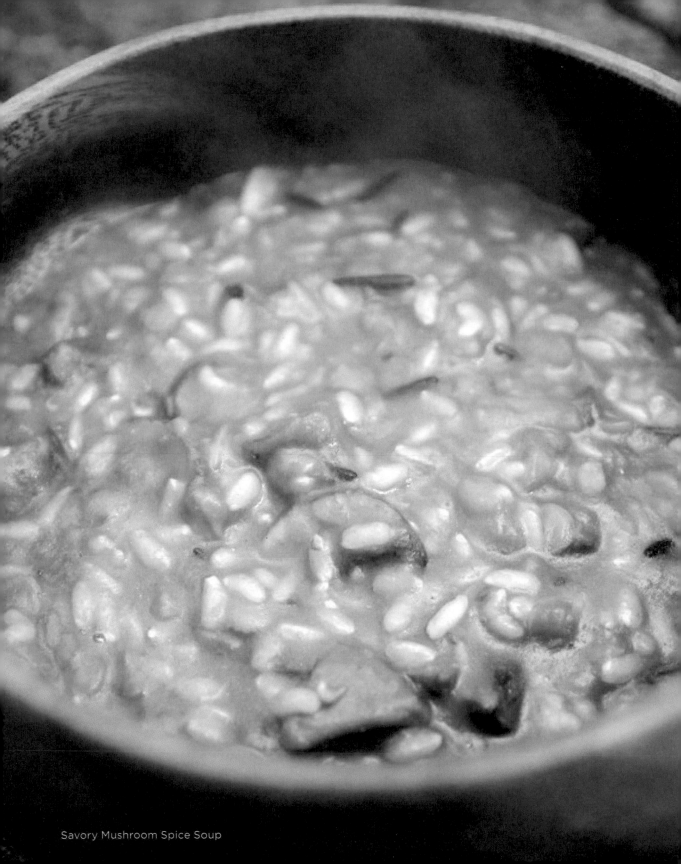

Savory Mushroom Spice Soup

SLURP IT

Having a nurturing, delicious bowl of hot soup for me is as comforting as soaking in a hot bath. The process of making soup is as healing and enjoyable as savoring every last spoonful. I love playing in the kitchen, inventing new recipes, trying out daring combinations of veggies and spices, and taste testing all the way. I feel like a pro when I add a dash of this and chop a bit more of that, tossing in the saucepan with charisma and flare. Good music and dancing around the kitchen always adds to the festivities. When you use great ingredients, you can't go too wrong. There have only been a few times where I made irreversible decisions in soup making, and it usually had to do with adding too many hot peppers, but I'll always tough it out and enjoy it anyway. The following are a few of my tested (don't worry) favorite go-to soups that I make all the time and that keep me feeling nurtured, cozy, and comforted, no matter what the day brings.

Pumpkin Coconut Cream Soup

PUMPKIN COCONUT CREAM SOUP

Fall is my favorite season. I love big fuzzy sweaters, cozy knitted hats, getting lost on long walks, and playing in the leaves. I love the crisp, fresh smell in the air, the bright blue skies, and the transition of the greens of summer to a rainbow of reds, yellows, and browns. Plus, in the fall, we are blessed with nature's nutrients from pumpkins, squash, tomatoes, corn, potatoes, and more. Growing up, we had so many buckets full of vegetables from our garden that my mom and grandma would prepare all we could eat and then can and store the rest for the winter. I am reminded of these things each fall, and this time of abundance always makes me remember to be thankful, prepare, and reflect. This pumpkin soup is like fall in a pot. I hope you love it as much as I do.

SERVES 4

1 small pumpkin, cut in half vertically

½ red onion, chopped

2 tablespoons olive oil

2 cups water

1 teaspoon red pepper flakes

1 teaspoon cinnamon

1 teaspoon nutmeg

1 teaspoon sea salt

1 teaspoon chili powder

½ cup coconut milk

2 tablespoons pumpkin seeds (optional)

1 tablespoon dried cranberries (optional)

Preheat the oven to 350 degrees Fahrenheit.

Scoop the seeds out of the pumpkin and roast it, cut sides down, in a pan for 40 minutes.

Scoop out the cooked pumpkin.

Sauté the onion until soft in the olive oil in a large soup pot.

Add the pumpkin and water to the pot.

Cover and simmer for 20 minutes.

Add the spices and simmer, covered, for 10 more minutes.

Stir in the coconut milk and simmer, covered, for 10 more minutes.

Blend the soup, transfer it to bowls, and top it with pumpkin seeds and dried cranberries, if desired.

ENJOY!

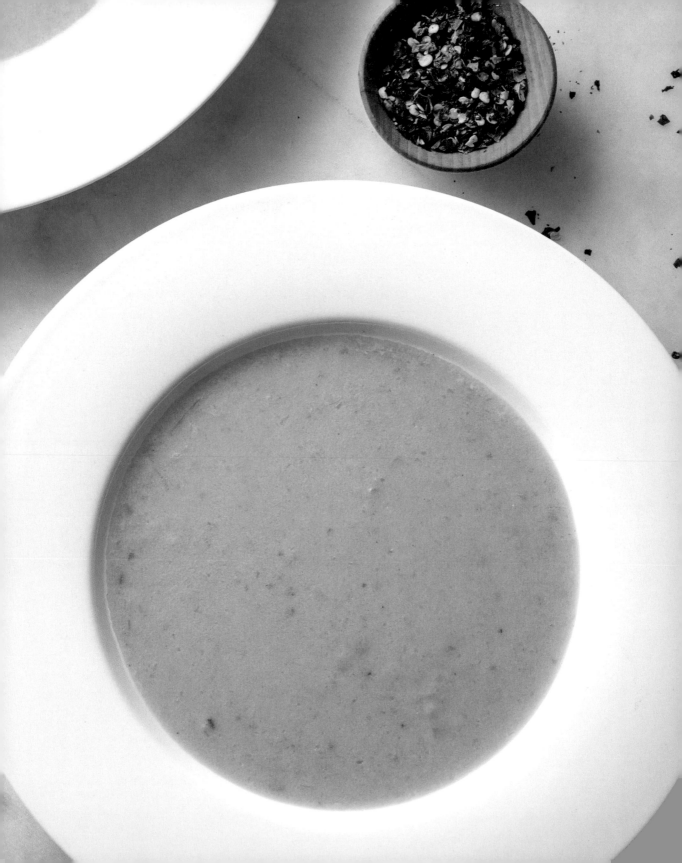

VEGGIE DETOX SOUP

I travel a lot, but when I know I am going to be home for at least a week, I love to cook up a big batch of this mouthwatering soup, which I invented a few winters ago when I got inspired to make all kinds of soups. I experimented with a bunch of fresh ingredients. I made some keepers, and some onetime adventures that weren't the best but were edible enough not to waste. The great thing about cooking with fresh ingredients is you can't go too far wrong. This soup is not only delicious; I've found that if I'm looking to clean out my system or recover from some travel tummy troubles, eating this soup for two out of three meals a day gets me back to having lots of energy, feeling lighter in my body, and being clear and calm in my mind.

SERVES 8

½ red onion, chopped

3 cloves garlic, minced

1 tablespoon olive oil

3 cups water or veggie stock

4 handfuls chopped veggies*

2 tablespoons hot sauce

1 teaspoon red pepper flakes

1 teaspoon black pepper

1 teaspoon curry powder

1 teaspoon chili powder

1 teaspoon sea salt

1 cup coconut milk

Sauté the onion and garlic in the olive oil in a large soup pot, until the onion is soft.

Add the water or veggie stock.

Stir in the veggies, hot sauce, and spices.

Bring the mixture to a boil, and then turn down to low and simmer for 30 minutes.

Stir in the coconut milk and simmer for 10 more minutes.

Enjoy blended or as is!

ENJOY!

*You can really use any vegetables that you like.
For me, I generally use a mixture of sweet potato, celery, cauliflower, tomato, and jalapeño.

SAVORY MUSHROOM SPICE SOUP

New York is filled with Asian-fusion restaurants, and I love so many of them. The idea of a warm bowl filled with spicy, savory goodness is a winner for me. I've experimented a lot with a spicy mushroom soup and gotten it way wrong many times. Too runny, too thick, too spicy, and too bland—I've messed up many batches along the way. It's been a long road, but I am happy to say that I finally created a recipe that works every time. I hope you enjoy it as much as I do.

SERVES 2

½ red onion, chopped

2 cloves garlic, minced

1 tablespoon extra-virgin olive oil

2 handfuls chopped cremini mushrooms

3 cups water

1 tablespoon red curry paste

1 tablespoon hot sauce

1 teaspoon red pepper flakes

Salt and pepper, to taste

½-inch ginger, peeled and minced

Juice of ¼ lemon

2 tablespoons cornstarch

1 cup mixture lentils and rice, cooked

Sauté the onion and garlic in the olive oil in a large soup pot, until the onion is soft.

Add the mushrooms and water.

Cover and simmer for 10 minutes.

Stir in the curry paste, hot sauce, red pepper flakes, salt and pepper, ginger, and lemon juice.

Cover and simmer for 10 more minutes.

Mix in the cornstarch, cover, and simmer for 10 more minutes.

When soup thickens, stir in the lentils and rice.

ENJOY!

TOMATO CREAM SOUP

When I first moved to New York, my diet consisted of way too much canned tomato soup. It was easy, and it filled me up. Thankfully I learned along the way that eating something that tasted okay and getting full wasn't all there was to eating. I still love tomato soup, but, since my canned soup days are long behind me, I've figured out my own concoction of healthy and savory goodness. I hope you enjoy this version as much as I do.

SERVES 4

4 organic tomatoes
2 cloves garlic, minced
1 red onion, chopped
1 tablespoon olive oil
1 red bell pepper, chopped
1 teaspoon red pepper flakes
¼ cup coconut milk

Preheat the oven to 350 degrees Fahrenheit.

Place the whole tomatoes and half of the garlic in a pan, and roast them for 15 to 20 minutes.

Meanwhile, sauté the onion and remaining garlic in the olive oil in a saucepan, until onion is soft.

After the tomatoes have cooled a bit, chop them and add them and the roasted garlic to saucepan.

Stir in the red bell pepper and the red pepper flakes.

Cover and simmer for 20 minutes.

Stir in the coconut milk, cover, and simmer for 10 more minutes.

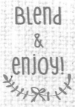

BLEND
&
ENJOY!

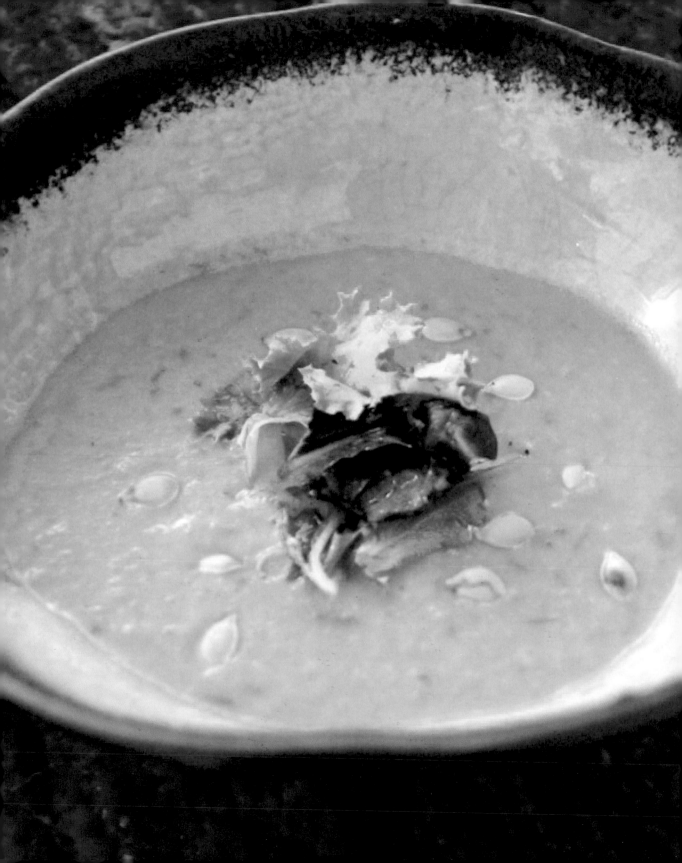

ROASTED ACORN SQUASH SOUP

Roasted Acorn Squash Soup can warm you deep down inside on a cold day.
Squash are supereasy to find in the fall and fun to pick up at your local farmers' market or grocery, and put you right in harvest mode.

SERVES 4

1 acorn squash, cut in half vertically

½ red onion, chopped

2 tablespoons olive oil

1 red pepper, chopped

2 cups water

½ cup almond milk

2 tablespoons pumpkin seeds (optional)

Preheat the oven to 350 degrees Fahrenheit.

Scoop the seeds out of the squash and roast it, cut sides down in a pan, for 40 minutes.

Scoop out the cooked squash.

In a large soup pot, sauté the onion until soft in the olive oil.

Add the squash, red pepper, and water to the pot.

Cover and simmer for 20 minutes.

Stir in the almond milk, and simmer, covered, for 10 more minutes.

Transfer it to bowls, and top with pumpkin seeds.

ENJOY!

FORK IT

When I was growing up, going out to eat was kind of a big deal. It was something we did on special occasions or if we were far away from home. We all agreed that home cooking was much healthier and tastier, but sometimes it was fun or necessary to go out. Salad bars were something that have stuck in my head from that time, mainly the experience of being just tall enough to see over the sneeze guard and peek into all the different dishes displayed. I used to fill my plate with a smorgasbord of spinach, beans, and Jell-O salad. While the adults viewed salad as something that goes on the side of the plate, in a fraction of the real estate that meat and potatoes demand, I believed in the potential and fun that can be gained from salads as the main event.

Now that I'm all grown up, big salads for meals are something that all reasonable, healthy adults view as a normal part of the day. Loaded up with color, the more variety, the better, salads as the main event are the way to go. Now there are chain restaurants all over the world dedicated to creating your own salad. I knew I had my finger on the pulse when I was tiptoeing up to that sneeze guard to investigate. Put away your tiny salad bowls and bring out your giant serving dishes for these bad boys. Salads are taking center stage!

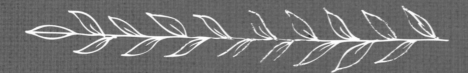

CHOPT & SPICY

I discovered the Chopt & Spicy one day when I was pretty hungry. I had a ton of fruits and veggies in my house, but no rice, pasta, or heartier bites that I generally turn to when I'm feeling famished. So I did what I could. I tossed a bunch of veggies in a bowl and combined them with a creamy, healthy dressing. And without planning it, I created a salad that I make all the time—because it's such a satisfying meal.

SERVES 2

¼ fresh pineapple, chopped
1 avocado, chopped
1 orange bell pepper, chopped
4 handfuls spinach, chopped
2 tablespoons balsamic vinegar
2 teaspoons Dijon mustard
Red pepper flakes, to taste

Combine pineapple, avocado, bell pepper, and spinach in a big bowl.
Mix the balsamic vinegar, Dijon mustard, and red pepper flakes to create the dressing in a separate bowl.
Toss the dressing with the fruits and vegetables.

ENJOY!

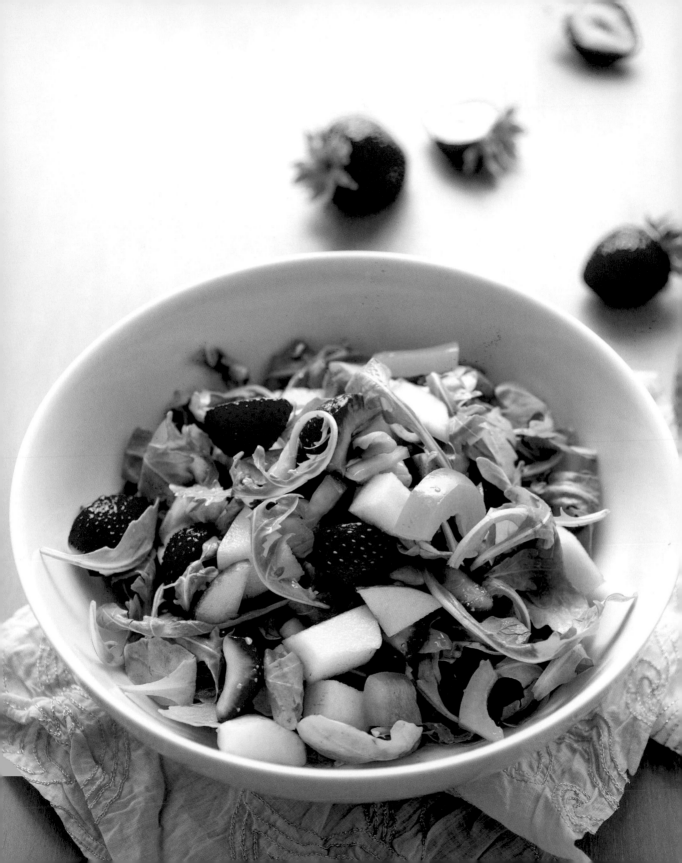

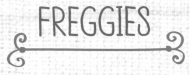

FREGGIES

The food-combining police might come after me for mixing fruits and veggies in this purposeful combination, but after I discovered Freggies one day, I never looked back. The combination of sweet strawberries, tart apples, bitter arugula, and savory cashews is a party in the mouth that leads to a satisfied belly.

SERVES 2

5 strawberries, chopped
½ apple, any variety, chopped
1 handful arugula
1 orange bell pepper, chopped
½ cucumber, chopped
¼ cup chopped cashews
Juice of ½ lime*

Mix all ingredients in a large bowl.

ENJOY!

*If you'd like a creamier dressing, mix a little balsamic vinegar and Dijon mustard with the lime juice.

MUSHROOM MADNESS

It's not really fair to call this salad a salad. It's more like a supermeal.

Hearty mushrooms and crunchy celery, combined with rice, lentils, avocado, and a few special surprises, create a dish that you will love. You won't be wanting anything more with this bad boy!

SERVES 2

5 cremini mushrooms, chopped

2 stalks celery, chopped

1 avocado, chopped

1 handful mixed greens, chopped

1 tablespoon nutritional yeast

½ cup mixture lentils and rice, cooked

2 tablespoons balsamic vinegar

2 teaspoons Dijon mustard

2 shakes of hot sauce

Mix together the mushrooms, celery, avocado, greens, and nutritional yeast in a large bowl.

Fold in the lentil and rice mixture.

Combine the balsamic vinegar, Dijon mustard, and hot sauce in a small bowl, whisking until smooth to create the dressing.

Add the dressing to the veggie mixture, and stir until it's evenly dispersed.

ENJOY!

KALE KRUNCH

We know by now how awesome kale is for us. Whether you are already on a healthy path or just beginning your journey, kale is here to stay. That doesn't mean it has to get tired, old, and boring. I try to get a lot of kale in my diet because I know the power of the super green, but it has to be yummy and exciting; otherwise I'm not interested. Whether you eat kale plain or like it dressed up, this salad will keep the healthy party going all night long.

SERVES 2

1 handful kale, broken up into manageable pieces
Juice of 1 lemon
1 orange bell pepper, chopped
2 stalks celery, chopped
Juice of 1 lime

Place the kale in a large bowl, and drizzle lemon juice over it.
Massage the kale–lemon juice mixture until it shrinks up a bit, about 2 minutes.
Mix in the pepper and celery.
Drizzle lime juice over the mixture, and mix it with your hands.

ENJOY!

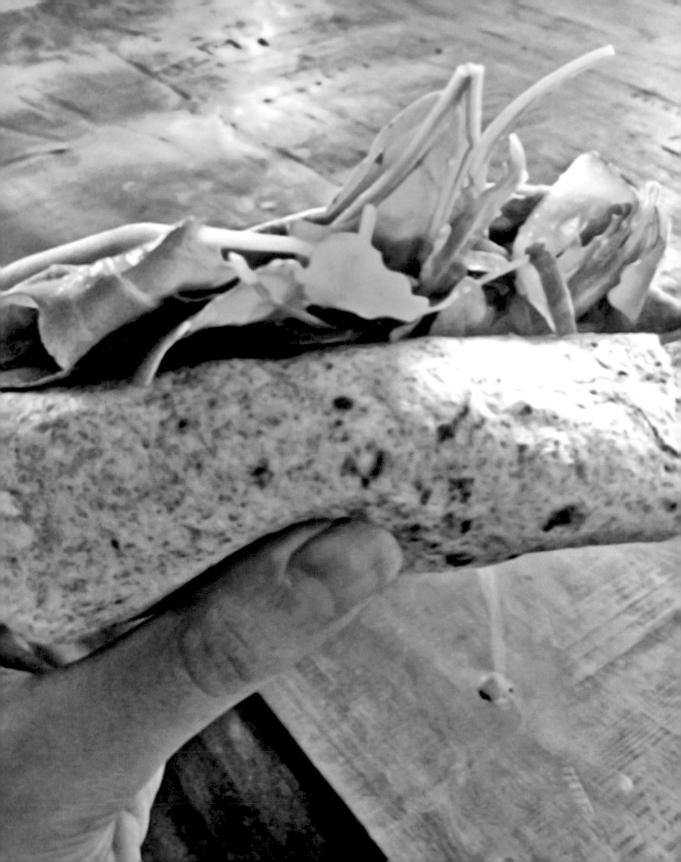

WRAP IT UP

I never really noticed wraps being a thing outside of the soft shell tacos that my mom whipped up occasionally when I was a kid. Maybe wraps as we know them now weren't invented yet. They weren't as popular as they are today, for sure. In NYC you can walk by any deli or sandwich shop and pick up a variety of mystery wraps with a vast difference in quality and taste. Wraps have gotten a bad rap I think, because of the secrets that can be hidden within. You think it's possibly good for you because there are some vegetables in there, but it is really loaded up with Thousand Island dressing and it turns out it's healthier to eat a bucket of French fries.

I admit, I've tried dozens of mystery wraps over the years, and mostly I felt pretty awful afterward. I would either get a burst of energy and then crash, just like from a bag of Sour Patch Kids, or I would feel sluggish right way and want to nap all afternoon. I appreciate the wrap, and I want to love the wrap, so there has to be a better way.

We can change their reputation by making our own at home! One of my favorite things about cooking is that you know exactly what you are eating because you are preparing everything.

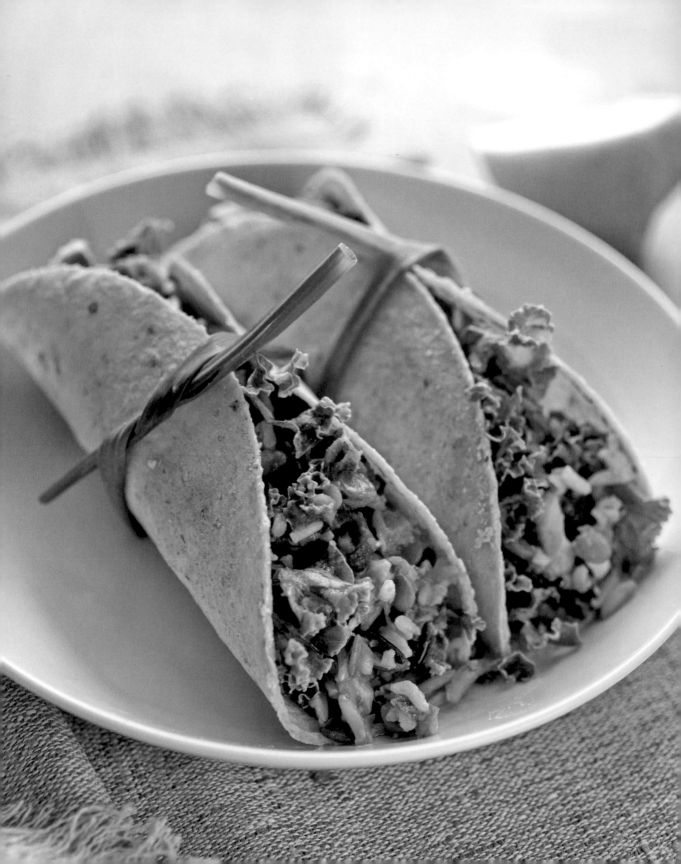

MEXICAN CHILLED WRAP

This Mexican Chilled Wrap is one of the first wraps I played around with at home and found worked for me. It reminds me of the soft shell tacos my mom used to make. It is an updated version with loads of tasty ingredients. It's satisfying and leaves you with gobs of energy and inspiration. It's great for a quick lunch at home or on the go.

SERVES 2

1 handful kale, torn into manageable pieces
Juice of 1 lemon
5 black or green olives
1 handful arugula
2 tablespoons salsa
½ cup guacamole (page 197)
½ cup mixture lentils and rice, cooked
4 corn tortillas

Place the kale in a large bowl, and drizzle lemon juice over it.
Massage the kale-lemon juice mixture until it shrinks up a bit, about 2 minutes.
Fold in the olives, arugula, salsa, guacamole, and lentils and rice.
Warm the tortillas in a skillet for 30 seconds.
Wrap the vegetable mixture in the tortillas.

ENJOY!

ALL VEGGIES IN MY BURRITO

I love to eat this burrito when I feel like I need a good dose of veggies but am craving something with more warmth and bite than a big salad. You can use pretty much any veggie you can imagine, but this is the combo I generally stick with. And I love the substitution of quinoa here for rice for that extra superfood punch.

SERVES 2

½ cup quinoa, cooked
½ cup canned black beans, drained and rinsed
1 cup broccoli, steamed
1 handful spinach, steamed
1 tomato, chopped
2 tablespoons salsa
Juice of 1 lime
4 corn or wheat tortillas

Combine the quinoa, black beans, broccoli, spinach, tomato, and salsa in cast-iron skillet over medium heat.
Stir and simmer until warm, about 5 minutes.
Squeeze fresh lime juice over entire mixture.
Wrap it up.

ENJOY!

HUMMUS CITRUS QUINOA WRAP

This hummus wrap cracks open a whole new arena of wraps. Often the wraps I discovered in delis were slapped with mystery goo that was supposed to give them some sort of flavor. What I've found is that adding hummus to the mix adds a ton of flavor, protein, and nutrients, and it removes the need for mystery goo.

SERVES 2

1 handful arugula
2 tablespoons hummus
1 red bell pepper, chopped
4 green and black olives
Juice of 1 lemon
4 corn or wheat tortillas

Mix together the arugula, hummus, pepper, and olives in a large bowl.
Toss the mixture with the lemon juice to coat.
Wrap it up.

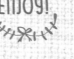

ENJOY!

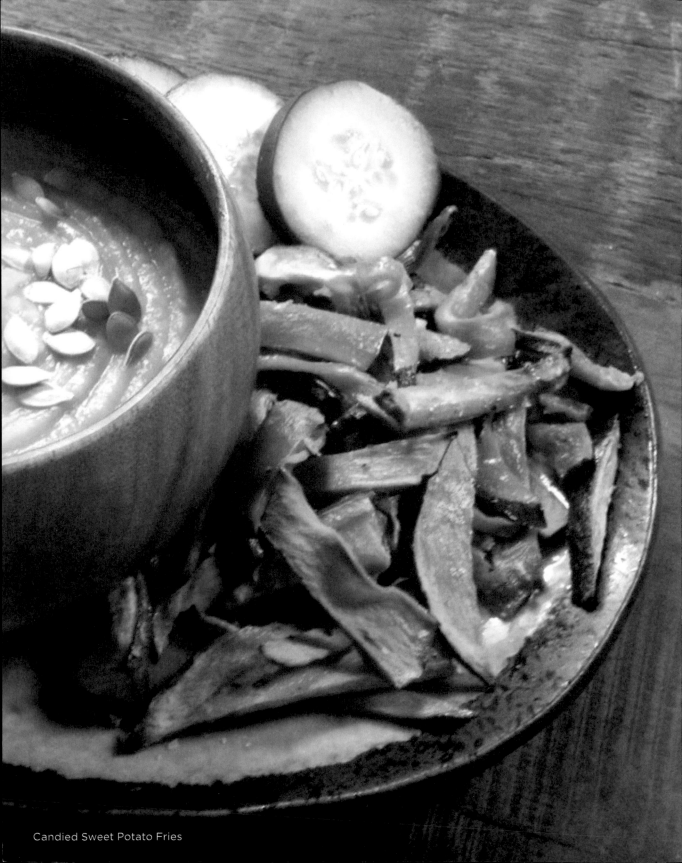

Candied Sweet Potato Fries

ON THE SIDE

When I think of side dishes, family reunions come to mind. Picnic areas filled with close and distant cousins, aunts, uncles, and grandparents—and everyone's Tupperware filled with their favorite side dishes. I had family members whose cooking I knew I could trust, and others whose skills were iffy at best. I remember a number of proclamations, such as "the best coleslaw in the world," not quite living up to the hype. Perhaps this is what started me on my make-your-own-rules path. Whenever adults tried to convince me to eat food that I wasn't instinctively interested in, I was suspicious. But, even as a child, I quickly learned that "Your Jell-O marshmallow salad looks gross!" was *not* a polite response.

The side dishes that have stuck with me are influenced by those people I did trust and by the comfort foods brought to all those family reunions. But now I've updated them so I can eat them as part of a healthy lifestyle that will keep me coming back to family reunions for as many years as possible. Now that it's my turn to show up with a side dish to contribute, I have some healthy favorites I can whip up on a moment's notice for any reunion—or even a quiet night at home.

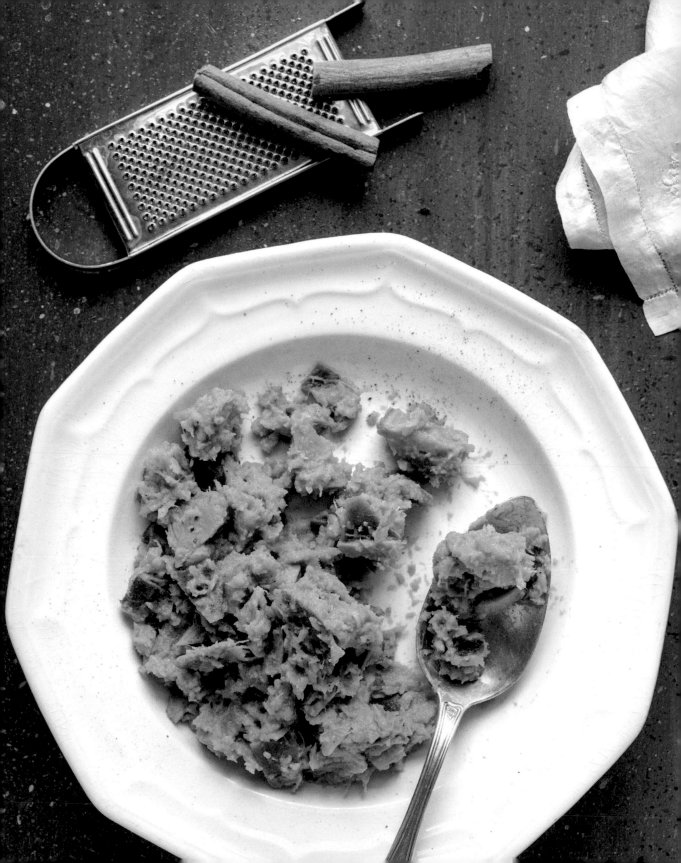

MASHED SWEET POTATOES

Mashed sweet potatoes are an absolute favorite side of mine. I'll eat them for breakfast or as a main dish if I'm not splitting them among a bunch of people. They are packed full of vitamins and are super yummy. I have an extrasweet and creamy version that I hope you love as much as I do.

SERVES 2

2 sweet potatoes, cubed
1½ teaspoons cinnamon
1 teaspoon nutmeg
1½ teaspoons nondairy buttery spread
2 tablespoons maple syrup
½ cup almond milk

Boil the sweet potatoes until tender, about 15 minutes.
Strain the potatoes and transfer them to a large bowl.
Mash the potatoes with a fork.
Add the remaining ingredients and stir until well combined.

ENJOY!

CANDIED SWEET POTATO FRIES

French fries could be an unhealthy habit if I let myself drift off into salt-and-sugar land, but fortunately I've discovered a homemade version that is equally decadent and nowhere near as destructive for the body, mind, and soul as the drive-through offering. When you make your own food instead of ordering it, you gain a whole new appreciation for yourself and for food without even trying. Mindless French fry consumption turns into appreciation of your creations and gratitude for the good fortune of having the resources and time to spend in the kitchen. You can check out a picture of these on page 220.

SERVES 2

2 sweet potatoes, thinly sliced
¼ cup coconut oil
½ cup maple syrup
Pinch of sea salt

Soak the sweet potatoes in water for 30 minutes, then drain them and dry them with a towel.

Preheat the oven to 350 degrees Fahrenheit.

Combine the sweet potatoes in a bowl with the coconut oil and maple syrup.

Mix until the sweet potatoes are thoroughly coated.

Place on cookie sheet and sprinkle with the sea salt.

Bake for 35 minutes, tossing the fries occasionally with a spatula to avoid burning.

Remove them from the oven, and let them cool a bit.

ENJOY!

STEAMED KALE WITH A KICK

Kale is king, and if you're able to get cozy with several kale recipes, you'll have no problem working it in on a regular basis. For me, adding some spice and some creamy flavor is all I need to convince me to down a bunch of the good stuff on the go. Stock up and enjoy!

SERVES 2

2 handfuls kale, steamed
4 shakes hot sauce
1 tablespoon nutritional yeast

Combine all ingredients.

ENJOY!

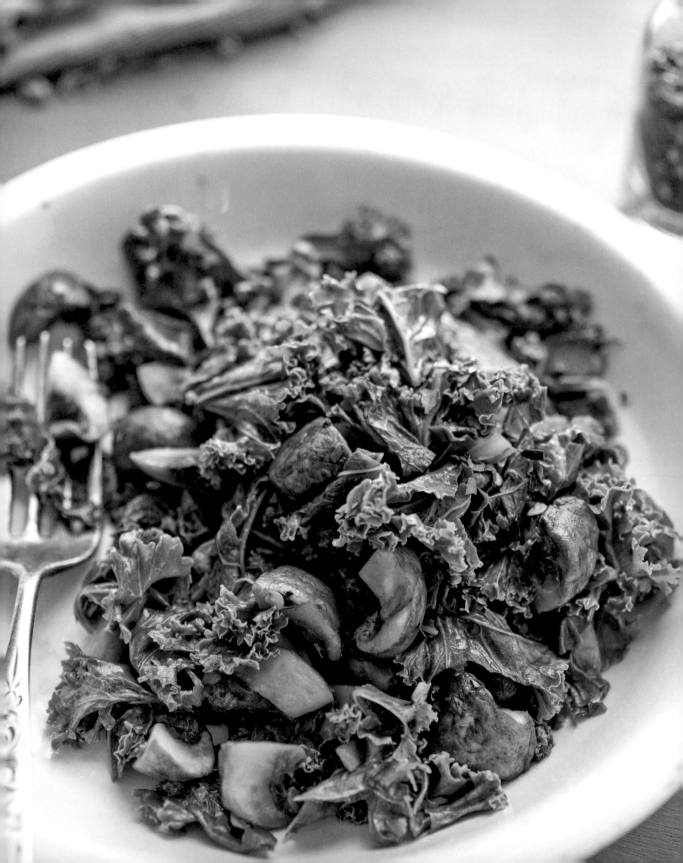

SPICY SAUTÉED MUSHROOM AND KALE

Getting mushrooms and kale together is a brawny powerhouse treat.

When spice is added, the flavors all dance together and present you with an impressive snack. I dare you to make this as a side for a dinner party or bring it to a potluck. It's so simple, but it's always a star.

SERVES 2

2 handfuls kale, torn into manageable pieces
Juice of 1 lemon
1 tablespoon nondairy buttery spread
5 cremini mushrooms, chopped
1½ teaspoons red pepper flakes
Pinch of sea salt

Combine the kale and lemon juice, and massage it until it shrinks, about 2 minutes.

Melt the nondairy buttery spread in a cast-iron skillet over medium heat.

Add the kale and mushrooms.

Stir for 5 minutes.

Transfer the mixture to a bowl and mix in the red pepper flakes and sea salt.

ENJOY!

SPINACH & QUINOA DELIGHT

Spinach and Quinoa Delight can only be categorized as one of those it's-so-simple-how-can-it-be-so-yummy dishes! A steamer and a few secret spices really go a long way. This is a great snack and so quick to make during a busy day that I often find myself whipping it up to eat as a whole meal. Or I pair it with another side—such as mashed sweet potatoes (page 223)—to give myself some variety and a beautiful plate.

SERVES 2

1 cup quinoa, cooked
2 handfuls spinach, steamed
Juice of 1 lime
Pinch of sea salt

Combine quinoa and spinach.
Mix with the lime juice, and add the sea salt.

ENJOY!

MAIN EVENT

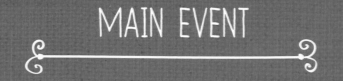

Lots of the recipes that can be served as side dishes can also be served as a stand-alone main event, but sometimes it's nice to have a few classic go-to meals in the repertoire to whip out when it's time to get dinner started. Following are a few of my favorites. I make these over and over, week after week, month after month. They never get old, and they are always great. I hope you enjoy my favorites, too!

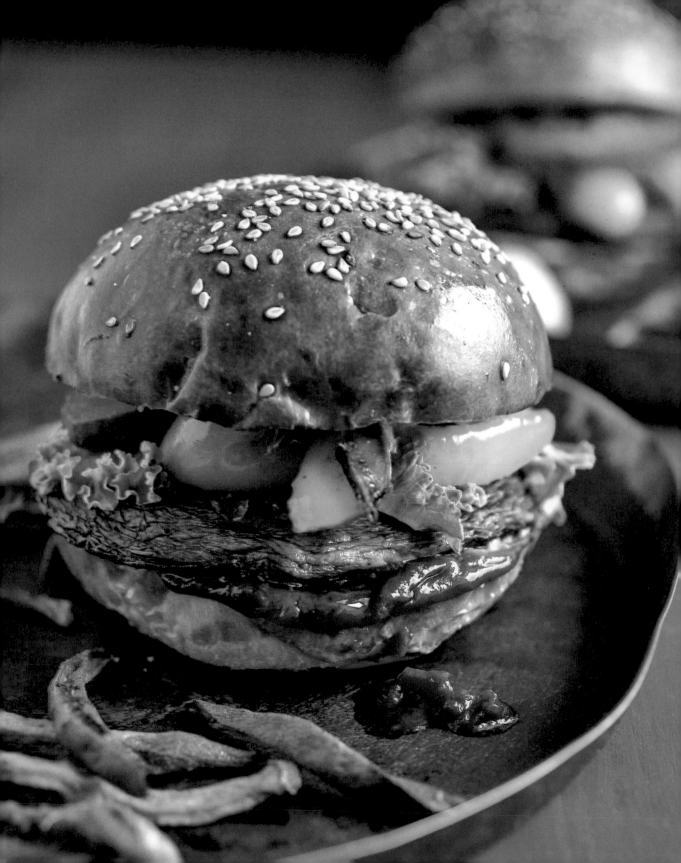

PORTOBELLO BURGER HEAVEN

This portobello burger is hearty, sweet, and savory. I have made these for a lot of people and have shared some of the information about how I get all the spice and flavor, but until now I haven't revealed everything because I like the burgers to be special and surprising. I'm psyched to share my secrets here with you, and I hope you enjoy them as much as I do.

SERVES 1

1 tablespoon olive oil
Pinch of sea salt
1 portobello mushroom
1½ teaspoons maple syrup
¼ tomato, sliced
½ orange or red bell pepper, sliced
Bun
Pickles, kale, organic ketchup, and Dijon mustard, to garnish

Preheat the oven to 350 degrees Fahrenheit.

Drizzle the olive oil and salt on the portobello.

Dip the portobello in the maple syrup.

Place portobello on a cookie sheet and bake it for 10 minutes.

Put the tomato slice and pepper on top of the portobello and bake for another 15 minutes.

Toast the bun in the oven for 5 minutes, if desired.

Remove everything from the oven and assemble the burger, garnishing with pickles, kale, ketchup, and Dijon mustard as desired.

ENJOY!

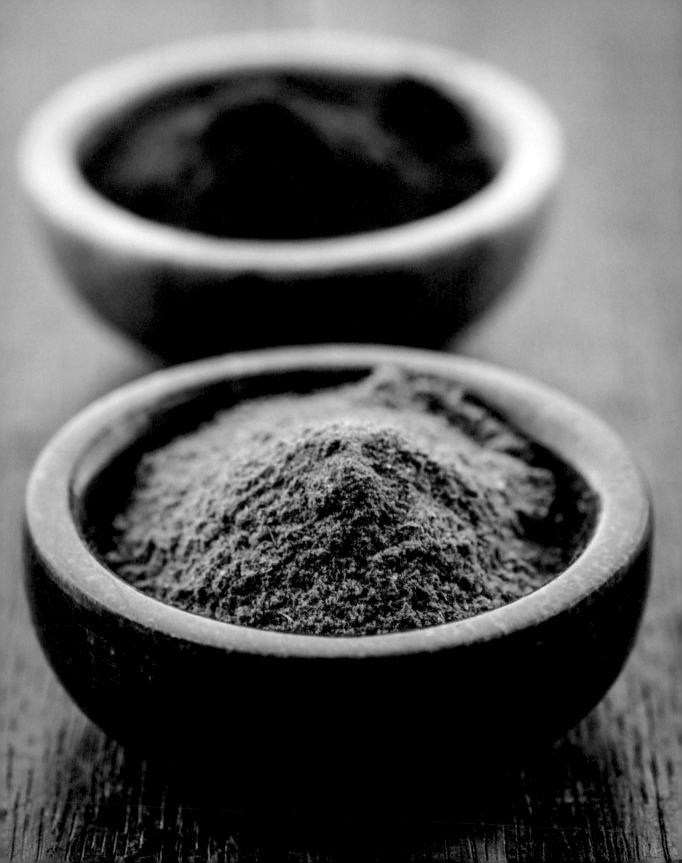

INDIAN CURRY MIX

When I'm in the mood for something with depth of flavor and staying power,
I turn to this Indian curry mix. It works with pretty much any vegetables that I have around. It's great to customize to what you have and what you love. This dish is great for a full, happy, and nourished belly.

SERVES 2

1 tablespoon nondairy buttery spread
2 stalks celery, chopped
2 carrots, chopped
2 handfuls kale, torn into manageable pieces
Juice of 1 lemon
2 cups mixture lentils and rice, cooked*
7 ounces nondairy curry sauce

Melt the nondairy buttery spread in a cast-iron skillet over medium heat.
Add the celery and carrots, and sauté until the vegetables are a little brown, about 5 minutes.
Add the kale, and continue to stir for 2 more minutes.
Drizzle the lemon juice on the mixture, then add the rice and lentils and the curry.
Continue to stir for 2 minutes.
Remove from the heat and transfer to serving bowls.

ENJOY!

*Quinoa is also delicious in this dish. Feel free to substitute.

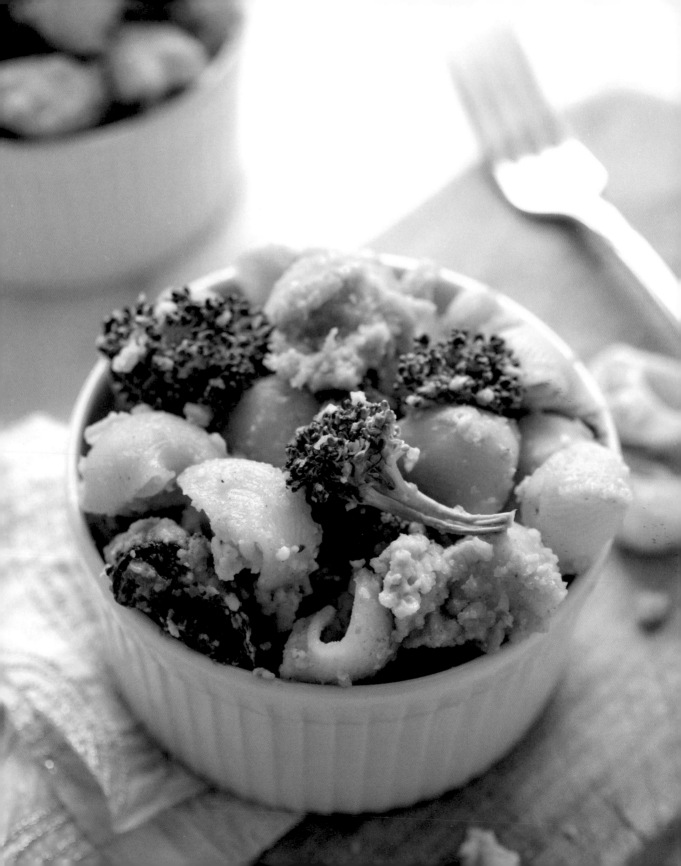

SHELLS & CHEESE

I grew up thinking cashews were a lesser nut, but now that I'm an adult, I'm totally into cashews and all the amazing ways they can be prepared and combined to make creamy goodness!

Not only are they delicious; they're really healthy. They have a lower fat content than most nuts, and most of their fat content is unsaturated fat, including oleic acid, the same monounsaturated fat in olive oil. Cashews are also magically healing. Studies have shown eating cashews can reduce your colon cancer risk. They are a great source of antioxidants that protect from heart disease, and they boast a ton of magnesium and copper, which are great for strong bones and flexible joints.

Luckily, one of my favorite meals from childhood can be re-created using these healthy nuts rather than dairy. I learned about substituting cashews blended up with delicious spices for cheese sauce from an awesome food blog, detoxinista.com. I adapted her mac and cheese recipe to make it easy and repeatable for me. I make and eat this pretty much every week that I'm in my kitchen.

SERVES 4

4 cups pasta shells*
2 cups chopped broccoli
1 cup whole cashews
1 tablespoon Dijon mustard
½ cup water

1½ teaspoons red pepper flakes
1 teaspoon curry powder
½ cup nutritional yeast
2 cups chopped cremini mushrooms
Juice of ½ lemon

Preheat the oven to 350 degrees Fahrenheit.
Prepare the pasta according to package directions.
Meanwhile, spread the broccoli on a cookie sheet and place it into the oven
    until the tops are browned, approximately 15 to 20 minutes.
Blend cashews, Dijon mustard, water, red pepper flakes, curry powder, and
    nutritional yeast in a blender until smooth to create the sauce.
When the pasta is tender, remove it from the heat and drain.
Put the pasta back into the pot, and add the broccoli, mushrooms, and sauce.
Stir the mixture until fully combined.
Pour the entire mixture into a glass baking dish.
Bake for 25 minutes.
After removing the pasta from the oven, drizzle with the lemon juice.

ENJOY!

*You can also make this with quinoa, spaghetti squash, or really any type of pasta you'd like.

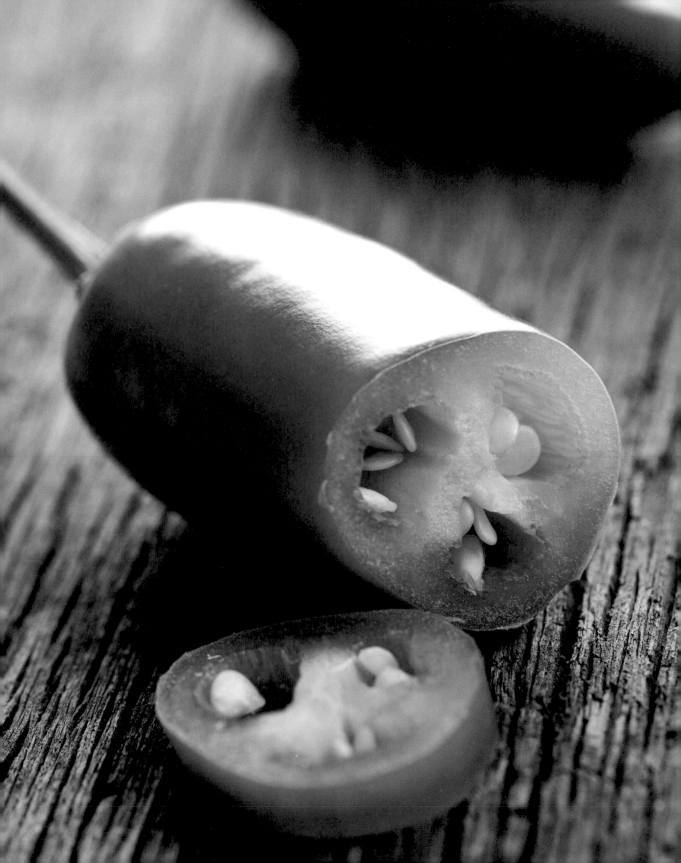

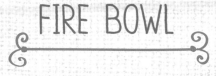

FIRE BOWL

Not long ago, the Buddha Bowl concept started popping up at healthy restaurants everywhere. It was like this ultimate warm bowl of healthy comfort food just landed on the planet and started taking over. I tried many of these bowls at several health food restaurants with friends, and the main thing I learned was that I love the concept, but often I dislike the execution. Too often I'd be picking around things I wasn't crazy about and not exactly loving the spices and flavors. So I decided to make my own. The Fire Bowl is one of my favorite combinations—but, as always, feel free to substitute ingredients to make it your own.

SERVES 2

½ red onion, chopped
1 tablespoon olive oil
2 cloves garlic, minced
1 red bell pepper, chopped
1 orange bell pepper, chopped
½ jalapeño pepper, chopped
½ cup canned black beans, drained and rinsed
½ cup mixture lentils and rice, cooked
Juice of 1 lime

Sauté onion in olive oil in a cast-iron skillet over medium heat for a few minutes until soft.

Toss in the garlic, and stir for a few more minutes.

Add the bell peppers and jalapeño, and continue to stir for a few more minutes.

Stir in the black beans and rice and lentils.

Continue to sauté the mixture for 5 to 10 more minutes, stirring continuously.

Remove from the heat, transfer to serving bowls, and drizzle with the lime juice.

ENJOY!

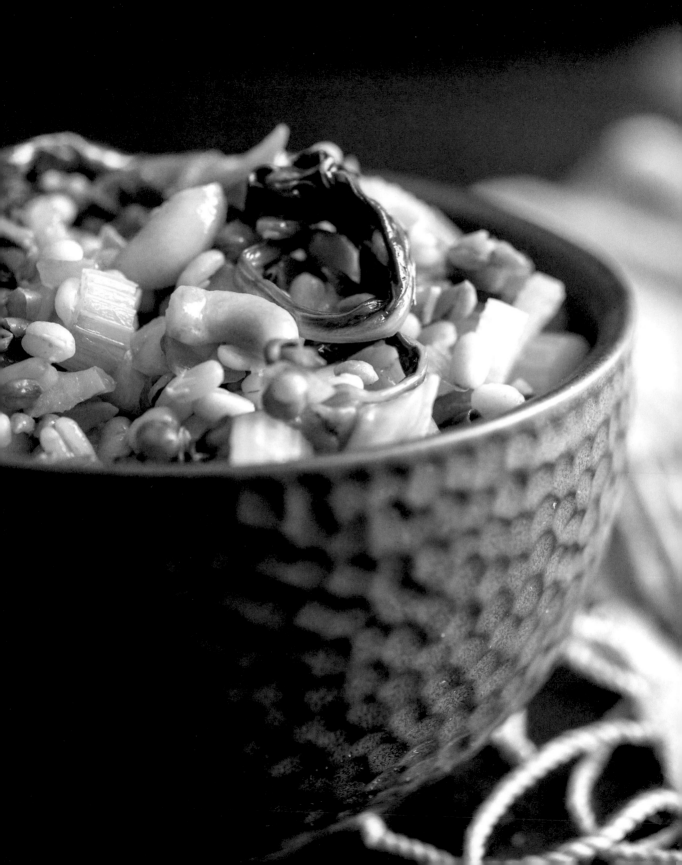

ENERGY BOWL

The Energy Bowl lives up to its name. Everything in this meal packs nutritional sustainability for the long haul. You'll feel jazzed up and ready for anything after one of these. Mung beans are a superfun discovery. They are simple and quick to make, and they leave you feeling awesome. I made this for friends once, and they said that they felt as if they had consumed energy and joy. Awesome.

SERVES 2

¼ red onion, chopped
1 tablespoon olive oil
2 stalks celery, chopped
1 cup cremini mushrooms, chopped
½ red bell pepper, chopped
1 handful spinach, chopped
½ cup whole cashews
1 cup mung beans, cooked
Juice of 1 lime

Sauté onion in olive oil in a cast-iron skillet over medium heat for 5 minutes, stirring regularly.

Add the celery, mushrooms, and pepper, and continue to stir for 5 more minutes.

Add the spinach and cashews and stir for 5 more minutes.

Add the mung beans and stir for 2 more minutes.

Remove from the heat, transfer to serving bowls, and drizzle with the lime juice.

ENJOY!

CHEESY KALE RICE

This dish will satisfy any need for creamy, rich pasta, but it doesn't leave you with the post-pasta tired feeling. The mixture of cheesy nutritional yeast with the rice, kale, and spices leaves your taste buds and belly superhappy. I like to make this after a long day of adventures when I'm in the mood for something rich and rewarding.

SERVES 2

1 cup wild rice
2 handfuls kale, torn into manageable pieces
Juice of 1 lemon
½ cup nutritional yeast
1 teaspoon sea salt
1 teaspoon red pepper flakes

Prepare the rice, adding a little water to the pot after rice is removed.
Steam the kale in the same pot.
Add the kale to the rice.
Stir in fresh lemon juice.
Stir in the nutritional yeast, sea salt, and red pepper flakes.

ENJOY!

INDULGE IT

I want to clear up one myth right now. Living healthy, eating well, and being radiant from the inside out has nothing to do with depriving yourself. A life without indulgence is a life without joy. Indulging in the sweet things of life—desserts and other adventures—reminds us that we are here to enjoy ourselves. Out of that simple diversion of joy, creativity thrives. Creativity is limitless, and it's the fuel we need to create meaningful things that help others find joy in life. When we quash our joy and try to do all the right things and live correctly, we not only put ourselves in a box, but we miss out on all the fun that fuels our passion. Give yourself the gift of your joy and indulge!

The following are some of my favorite desserts. I hope they bring you as much joy as they have brought me. Make your favorites for your friends so the joy can keep on radiating!

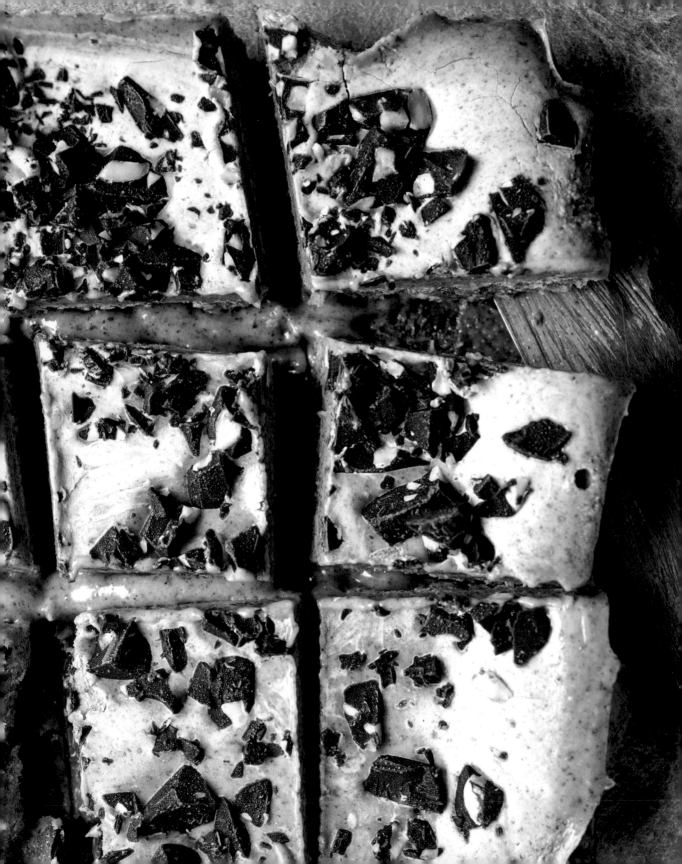

ALMOND BUTTER FUDGE

I make this treat weekly to have around as a snack and a dessert. Anytime guests come over it's a simple thing to whip up and always a huge hit. Like the Shells & Cheese (page 235), I adapted this recipe from detoxinista.com. I actually play around with the ingredients a lot, making it with peanut butter, chocolate peanut butter, or cashew butter, and topping it with all sorts of different chocolate treats. And it's always amazing! The combinations never get old, and it only takes three minutes to make . . . the freezer does the rest!

SERVES 8

¼ cup coconut oil
1 cup of almond butter*
1 tablespoon raw honey (optional)
½ teaspoon sea salt
1 handful dark chocolate chips
1 handful crushed dark chocolate bar

Soften the coconut oil by setting the container in a bowl of warm water for a few minutes.

Mix together the coconut oil, almond butter, honey, salt, and dark chocolate chips in a large bowl.

Pour the mixture into a glass dish lined with plastic wrap.

Top with the crushed chocolate bar.

Freeze the fudge for at least an hour.

Cut up in squares and serve.

Make sure to store the remaing fudge in the freezer.

ENJOY!

*You can use any kind of nut butter to make this. I've used all sorts.

APPLE CRISP

I have fond memories of a healthy version of apple crisp my mom used to bake on special occasions. It popped into my mind one day and onto my taste buds, and I had to have it immediately. I didn't have a ton of ingredients in the house that day, so I worked with what I had and it turned out so well that I make my own version on special occasions now!

SERVES 2

2 heaping tablespoons almond butter

1½ teaspoons coconut oil

2 tablespoons maple syrup

2 teaspoons cinnamon

2 honeycrisp apples (or any apples you love), chopped

Preheat the oven to 350 degrees Fahrenheit.

Mix together the almond butter, coconut oil, maple syrup, and cinnamon in a large bowl.

Add the apples and stir until evenly coated.

Pour the mixture into a glass baking dish.

Bake for 20 minutes.

Remove from the oven and let cool a bit before serving.

ENJOY!

PEANUT BUTTER COOKIE BARS

Sometimes you want a cookie, and sometimes it's nice to have a cookie bar.
I whipped up these peanut butter cookie bars with a lot of trial and error. It's an exciting moment when you find the perfect consistency, thickness, and chewiness to create a dessert that melts in your mouth. Cookie bar heaven emerges.

SERVES 6

2 cups almond or oat flour
2 tablespoons egg replacers
1 teaspoon baking soda
1 cup peanut butter*
½ cup maple syrup
½ cup coconut oil

Preheat the oven to 350 degrees Fahrenheit.
In a large bowl, mix everything together.
Pour the mixture into a glass baking dish.
Bake for 20 to 25 minutes, testing for doneness with a fork—the way you would test a cake.

ENJOY!

*You can also use almond butter in this recipe—or go crazy and use white chocolate peanut butter. I've done it, and it's yummy!

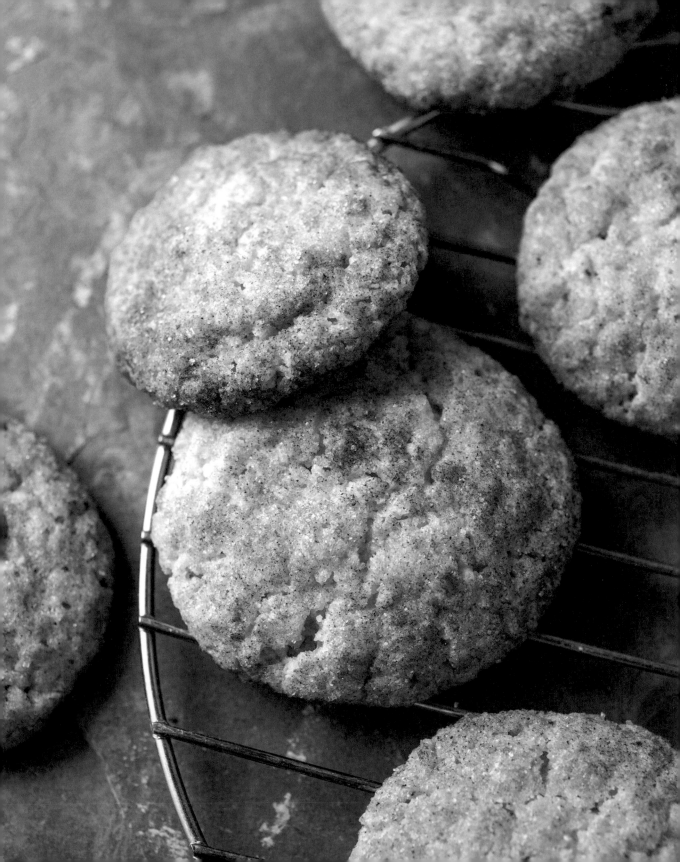

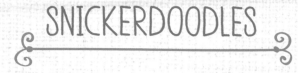
SNICKERDOODLES

Snickerdoodles are my all-time favorite cookie to make, to share with friends, and to eat. This love started when I could barely reach the counter. My aunt Sharron started a tradition in which my cousin Shelah and I got to roll the dough and cover the cookie balls in cinnamon and sugar. We had our assembly line down like pros and were always excited to enjoy our creations and share with friends and family. After some experimenting, I figured out a version to make that is a little healthier than our childhood version. Both versions are great, but I feel better about enjoying the updated one more often.

SERVES 6

1¾ cups all-purpose flour

¼ cup cornstarch

1 teaspoon baking powder

1 stick (4 ounces) nondairy butter

1¼ cups sugar

¼ cup vanilla almond milk

1 teaspoon vanilla extract

3 tablespoons cinnamon

Preheat the oven to 350 degrees Fahrenheit.

Whisk together flour, cornstarch, and baking powder in a bowl.

Use a hand mixer to beat the nondairy butter and ¾ cup of the sugar in a separate bowl until smooth.

Add the almond milk and vanilla extract and beat again until smooth.

Add the dry ingredients and beat until smooth.

Roll the dough into small even balls.

Mix together the remaining ½ cup sugar and the cinnamon in a small bowl.

Roll the dough balls in the cinnamon-sugar mixture.

Place the coated balls on a baking sheet, and bake for 15 to 20 minutes.

Remove from the oven, place on cooling rack, and let cool.

ENJOY!

BANANA SOFT SERVE

At one point, I heard a crazy rumor that you can turn bananas into ice cream. Apparently it just takes a frozen banana and a high-powered blender. No other ingredients are required. Now, I took this as a rumor because it seemed unlikely that a banana could ever be mistaken for ice cream unless it was mixed into a bowl of actual ice cream. But, since I'm always curious, I decided to give it a shot. I froze some bananas overnight. (Side note: make sure to peel your bananas before you freeze them because they are impossible to peel after frozen. Don't make the same mistakes as me!) The next day, I blended, and well…it was delicious. Now I make this a lot, and I add all sorts of things: chocolate, peppermint extract, almond butter. Anything you can imagine you'd like with your ice cream comes out fantastic. And it actually is fantastic all on its own. You have to experience this to believe it.

SERVES 2

3 frozen bananas, chopped
2 tablespoons cocoa powder*

Place bananas and cocoa powder in a high-powered blender.
Blend on the "frozen dessert" setting until it looks like ice cream.

ENJOY!

*Like I said, I've made this with all sorts of stuff. You can use 2 tablespoons of just about anything—I've even used hot chocolate powder.

ICE-CREAM SANDWICHES

I don't think I'll ever grow up, and that's just fine with me. Ice-cream sandwiches are a fun treat for all of us, no matter how young or old we are. Great when you're on your own or an impressive treat for guests. And to make these, I just combine two of my favorite desserts: Snickerdoodles (page 247) and Banana Soft Serve (page 248). It takes me right back to being a kid—but healthier.

SERVES 1

¼ cup Banana Soft Serve (page 248)
2 Snickerdoodles (page 247)

Put the soft serve between the cookies, and you have a winner!

ENJOY!

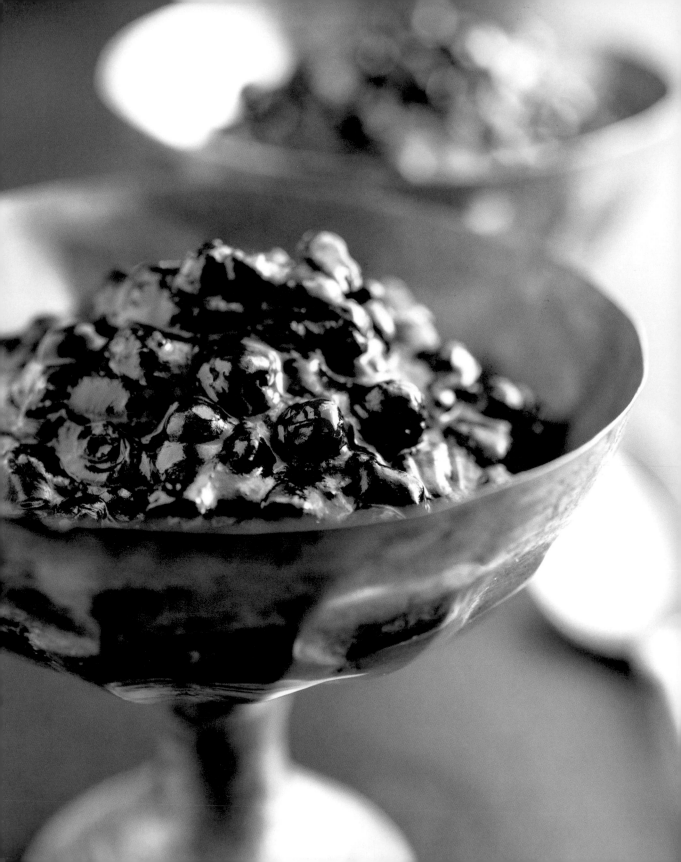

WARM CHOCOLATE BERRY BOWL

The ultimate comfort treat is a warm bowl of chocolate berry goodness.
I uncovered this delight one night after dinner. I was craving something warm and sweet and didn't have a lot of ingredients in the house. I found a bag of frozen mixed berries, a banana, and a dark chocolate bar and thought, *Hey, what happens if I warm it all up and mix it together?* I discovered a new favorite, ultimate, comfort sweet treat. I've served this one to guests, and it always makes for rave reviews and happy bellies.

SERVES 1

4 squares dark chocolate or ½ cup dark chocolate chips
1 banana, mashed
½ cup blueberries
1 teaspoon cinnamon

Combine the chocolate, banana, and blueberries in a saucepan over medium heat.
Stir constantly until chocolate and banana are melted.
Transfer to a bowl and top with cinnamon.

ENJOY!

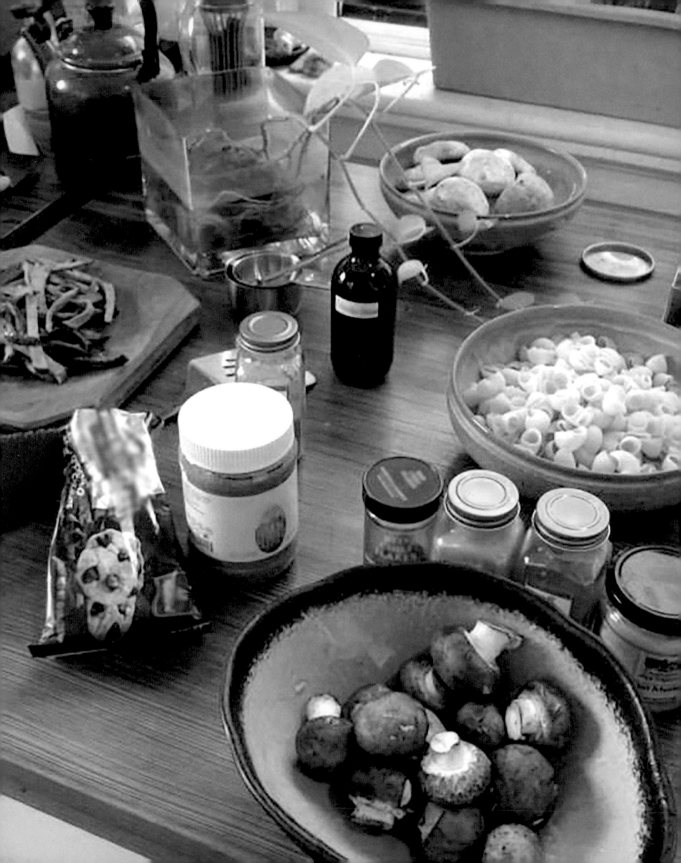

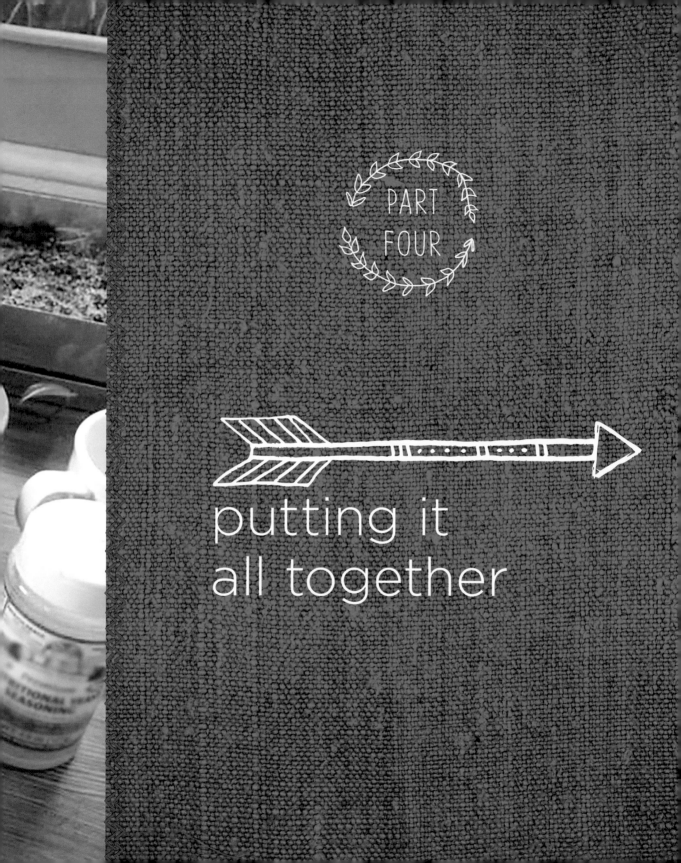

PART
FOUR

putting it
all together

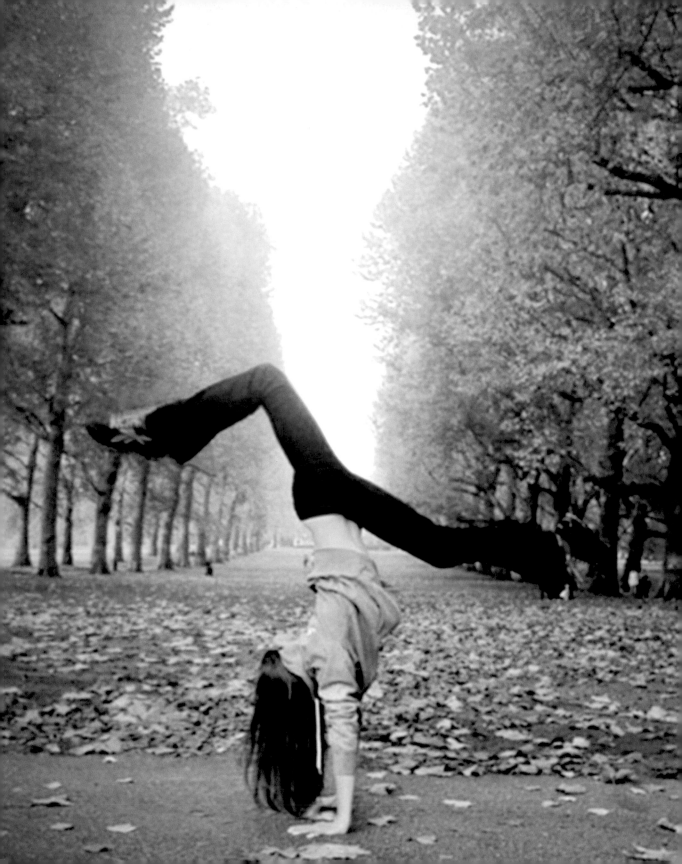

CHAPTER 9

7 days to radiate kick start

NOW it's time to put it all together and kick-start you on the road to radiance! If you don't feel like creating your own plan at this point, here's a seven-day schedule of meditation, yoga, and recipes you can use to leave you feeling calm, capable, and connected. Make sure to drink a lot of water throughout the day, as well. Get ready for transformation!

In general, you'll probably feel best if you don't eat a big meal right before you practice or too close to bedtime.

I like to give myself about an hour between eating a meal and practice. Having a smoothie, juice, or light snack such as a banana or some nuts about 20 minutes before a practice makes me feel energized. The most important thing to remember, however, is that this is all about you. Listen to your body. When you start to move more and practice regularly, you'll start to notice your preferences and how you feel. You might not want to eat right before you practice, or you may feel better if you have your juice or smoothie before you practice and breakfast after. When I began I found it helpful to keep a journal to note what I ate, when I ate, and how it made me feel. This really helped me get to know what was best for me, and I still keep one today.

DAY 1
Morning Meditation: two minutes of 4 Count Breathing (page 156), followed by three minutes of Alternate Nostril Breathing (page 156)
Breakfast: Maple French Toast (page 193) + Green River (page 170)
Yoga: Body Awareness Flow (page 107)
Lunch: Mexican Chilled Wrap (page 217)
Snack: Clementine Creamsicle (page 176)
Yoga: Easygoing Winding Down the Evening Flow (page 138)
Dinner: Energy Bowl (page 239) + Mashed Sweet Potatoes (page 223)
Dessert: Almond Butter Fudge (page 243)
Evening Meditation: Calm Eyes (page 162), followed by five minutes of Easy Breathing (page 155)

DAY 2

Morning Meditation: one minute of Breath of Fire (page 159), followed by four minutes of Mantra Meditation (page 160)

Breakfast: Granola (page 189) + The Popeye (page 172)

Yoga: Heart-Pumping Sweaty Flow (page 119)

Lunch: Freggies (page 211)

Snack: Spinach Cashew Mix (page 195)

Yoga: Easygoing Winding Down the Evening Flow (page 138)

Dinner: Cheesy Kale Rice (page 240)

Dessert: Peanut Butter Cookie Bars (page 245)

Evening Meditation: Hug the Universe (page 158) for two minutes

DAY 3

Morning Meditation: three minutes of Easy Breathing (page 155), followed by two minutes of Alternate Nostril Breathing (page 156)

Breakfast: The Swamp (page 181)

Yoga: Easy Mind Calm Body Flow (page 114)

Lunch: Kale Krunch (page 213)

Snack: Spinach and Quinoa Delight (page 228)

Yoga: Craving Control Flow (page 98)

Dinner: Shells & Cheese (page 235) + Chopt & Spicy (page 209)

Dessert: Banana Soft Serve (page 248)

Evening Meditation: three minutes of Bellows Breathing (page 160)

DAY 4
Morning Meditation: five minutes of Mantra Meditations (page 160)
Breakfast: Spicy Avocado Toast (page 191) + Turn Up the Beet (page 171)
Yoga: Energizing Morning Flow (page 80)
Lunch: Hummus Citrus Quinoa Wrap (page 219)
Snack: Strawberry Shortcake Smoothie (page 185)
Yoga: Body Awareness Flow (page 107)
Dinner: Portobello Burger Heaven (page 231) + Tomato Cream Soup (page 205)
Dessert: Warm Chocolate Berry Bowl (page 251)
Evening Meditation: five minutes of 4 Count Breathing (page 156)

DAY 5
Morning Meditation: one minute of Breath of Fire (page 159), followed by two minutes of Alternate Nostril Breathing (page 156)
Breakfast: All Veggies in My Burrito (page 218) + Green River (page 170)
Yoga: Craving Control Flow (page 98)
Lunch: Mushroom Madness (page 212)
Snack: Chocolate Almond Butter Protein Bomb (page 183)
Yoga: Easy Mind Calm Body Flow (page 114)
Dinner: Indian Curry Mix (page 233)
Dessert: Apple Crisp (page 244)
Evening Meditation: Calm Eyes (page 162)

DAY 6

Morning Meditation: five minutes of Easy Breathing (page 155)

Breakfast: Hot Fruit Bowl (page 190) + The Popeye (page 172)

Yoga: Energizing Morning Flow (page 80)

Lunch: Savory Mushroom Spice Soup (page 204)

Snack: Fresh Guacamole (page 197) with veggies

Yoga: Heart-Pumping Sweaty Flow (page 119)

Dinner: Shells & Cheese (page 235)

Dessert: Snickerdoodles (page 247)

Evening Meditation: three minutes of 4 Count Breathing (page 156)

DAY 7

Morning Meditation: one minute of Hug the Universe (page 158)

Breakfast: Spicy Avocado Toast (page 191) + Green River (page 170)

Yoga: Energizing Morning Flow (page 80)

Lunch: Pumpkin Coconut Cream Soup (page 201)

Snack: Savory & Spicy Mushroom Bites (page 196)

Yoga: Body Awareness Flow (page 107)

Dinner: Energy Bowl (page 239) + Mashed Sweet Potatoes (page 223)

Dessert: Ice-Cream Sandwiches (page 249)

Evening Meditation: one minute of Hug the Universe (page 158)

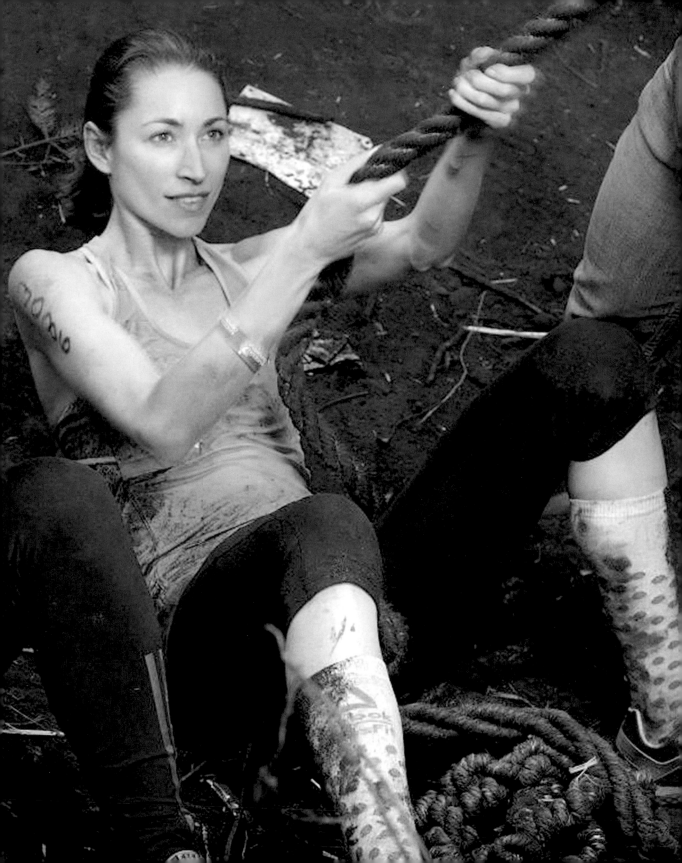

CHAPTER 10

30-day real-deal transformation plan

If you've done the seven-day kick start and want to keep going, but still don't want to create your own routine, here's one you can follow for 30 days. Not only will this transform you, but it will give you real-life experience and set you up to make your own rules for the rest of your days. Remember, this is about how you feel. So follow how you feel. Eat when you are hungry. Enjoy your meals and have fun practicing the yoga.

Feel free to substitute routines and recipes from the book if something fits more easily in your schedule, or you have the ingredients on hand for one recipe but not another. Drink plenty of water, and keep it with you during the day. If you are pressed for time, carry nuts and a piece of fruit for a snack.

Thirty days of meditating, practicing, and eating like this will have you feeling energetic and radiant from the inside out. Bonus benefits: your body will become leaner, stronger, and more open. Your skin will glow. You'll have more energy, feel less tired and sluggish, and have more creativity and freedom in your body, mind, and life.

I recommend keeping a journal throughout the 30 days. Document how you feel, what comes up in your yoga and meditation. Write down what recipes you love the most and any ideas you have to create your own. Document your dreams if you remember them, and write down how your energy levels are throughout the day. Any other creative thoughts that come up, write them down, too. You will probably be having loads of intuitive bursts during these next few weeks, so make sure to enjoy the ride! All of this will help you create the perfect rules for you as you move forward in your life.

DAY 1
Morning Meditation: five minutes of Easy Breathing (page 155)
Breakfast: Granola (page 189) (make a big batch for the week) + The Popeye (page 172)
Yoga: Body Awareness Flow (page 107)
Lunch: Veggie Detox Soup (page 203) (make a big batch for the week)
Snack: Steamed Kale with a Kick (page 225)
Yoga: Heart-Pumping Sweaty Flow (page 119)
Dinner: Energy Bowl (page 239)

Dessert: Almond Butter Fudge (page 243) (make a batch for the next few days)
Evening Meditation: three minutes of Bellows Breathing (page 160)
DAY 2
Morning Meditation: three minutes of Alternate Nostril Breathing (page 156)
Breakfast: The Swamp (page 181)
Yoga: Energizing Morning Flow (page 80)
Lunch: Veggie Detox Soup
Snack: Clementine Creamsicle (page 176)
Yoga: Easygoing Winding Down the Evening Flow (page 138)
Dinner: Fire Bowl (page 237)
Dessert: Almond Butter Fudge
Evening Meditation: Calm Eyes (page 162)
DAY 3
Morning Meditation: five minutes of Easy Breathing (page 155)
Breakfast: Granola + Green River (page 170)
Yoga: Heart-Pumping Sweaty Flow (page 119)
Lunch: Veggie Detox Soup
Snack: Healthy Frosty (page 178)
Yoga: Craving Control Flow (page 98)

Dinner: Mexican Chilled Wrap (page 217)
Dessert: Almond Butter Fudge
Evening Meditation: three minutes of 4 Count Breathing (page 156)
DAY 4
Morning Meditation: one minute of Breath of Fire (page 159)
Breakfast: Granola + Turn Up the Beet (page 171)
Yoga: Body Awareness Flow (page 107)
Lunch: Veggie Detox Soup
Snack: Spinach Cashew Mix (page 195)
Yoga: Craving Control Flow (page 98)
Dinner: Portobello Burger Heaven (page 231) + Mashed Sweet Potatoes (page 223)
Dessert: Snickerdoodles (page 247) (make a batch for the next couple of days—bring to work and share with friends, too)
Evening Meditation: Calm Eyes (page 162)
DAY 5
Morning Meditation: three minutes of Bellows Breathing (page 160)
Breakfast: Granola + The Popeye (page 172)
Yoga: Heart-Pumping Sweaty Flow (page 119)
Lunch: Veggie Detox Soup
Snack: Fresh Guacamole (page 197) with veggies
Yoga: Body Awareness Flow (page 107)

Dinner: Cheesy Kale Rice (page 240)
Dessert: Snickerdoodles
Evening Meditation: five minutes of Mantra Meditation (page 160)

DAY 6
Morning Meditation: three minutes of 4 Count Breathing (page 156)
Breakfast: Chocolate Almond Butter Protein Bomb (page 183)
Yoga: Body Awareness Flow (page 107)
Lunch: Chopt & Spicy (page 209)
Snack: Spinach and Quinoa Delight (page 228)
Yoga: Easy Mind Calm Body Flow (page 114)
Dinner: Indian Curry Mix (page 233)
Dessert: Apple Crisp (page 244) (make a batch for the next few days)
Evening Meditation: two minutes of Hug the Universe (page 158)

DAY 7
Morning Meditation: five minutes of Easy Breathing (page 155)
Breakfast: Hot Fruit Bowl (page 190)
Yoga: Heart-Pumping Sweaty Flow (page 119)
Lunch: Fire Bowl (page 237)
Snack: Savory & Spicy Mushroom Bites (page 196)
Yoga: Easy Mind Calm Body Flow (page 114)
Dinner: Savory Mushroom Spice Soup (page 204) (make a batch for the next few days)

Dessert: Apple Crisp
Evening Meditation: three minutes of Bellows Breathing (page 160)

DAY 8
Morning Meditation: one minute of Breath of Fire (page 159)
Breakfast: The Swamp (page 181)
Yoga: Energizing Morning Flow (page 80)
Lunch: Savory Mushroom Spice Soup
Snack: Clementine Creamsicle (page 176)
Yoga: Craving Control Flow (page 98)
Dinner: Spicy Sautéed Mushroom and Kale (page 227) + Mashed Sweet Potatoes (page 223)
Dessert: Apple Crisp
Evening Meditation: Calm Eyes (page 162)

DAY 9
Morning Meditation: five minutes of Mantra Meditation (page 160)
Breakfast: Maple French Toast (page 193) + Green River (page 170)
Yoga: Energizing Morning Flow (page 80)
Lunch: Mushroom Madness (page 212)
Snack: Spicy Avocado Toast (page 191)
Yoga: Easy Mind Calm Body Flow (page 114)
Dinner: Hummus Citrus Quinoa Wrap (page 219)
Dessert: Thin Mints Girl Scout Smoothie (page 179)
Evening Meditation: Calm Eyes (page 162)

DAY 10

Morning Meditation: five minutes of 4 Count Breathing (page 156)

Breakfast: Banango (page 177)

Yoga: Body Awareness Flow (page 107)

Lunch: Pumpkin Coconut Cream Soup (page 201) (make a batch for the next few days)

Snack: Creamy Eggless Nog (page 186)

Yoga: Easygoing Winding Down the Evening Flow (page 138)

Dinner: Kale Krunch (page 213) + Candied Sweet Potato Fries (page 224)

Dessert: Warm Chocolate Berry Bowl (page 251)

Evening Meditation: five minutes of Mantra Meditation (page 160)

DAY 11

Morning Meditation: five minutes of 4 Count Breathing (page 156)

Breakfast: Hot Fruit Bowl (page 190)

Yoga: Craving Control Flow (page 98)

Lunch: Pumpkin Coconut Cream Soup

Snack: Spinach Cashew Mix (page 195)

Yoga: Body Awareness Flow (page 107)

Dinner: All Veggies in My Burrito (page 218)

Dessert: Peanut Butter Cookie Bars (page 245) (make a batch for the next few days)

Evening Meditation: five minutes of Alternate Nostril Breathing (page 156)

DAY 12
Morning Meditation: one minute of Breath of Fire (page 159), followed by four minutes of Hug the Universe (page 158)
Breakfast: Maple French Toast (page 193) + Green River (page 170)
Yoga: Energizing Morning Flow (page 80)
Lunch: Pumpkin Coconut Cream Soup
Snack: Fresh Guacamole (page 197) with veggies
Yoga: Body Awareness Flow (page 107)
Dinner: Portobello Burger Heaven (page 231)
Dessert: Peanut Butter Cookie Bars
Evening Meditation: five minutes of Mantra Meditation (page 160)
DAY 13
Morning Meditation: Calm Eyes (page 162)
Breakfast: Banango (page 177)
Yoga: Body Awareness Flow (page 107)
Lunch: Tomato Cream Soup (page 205) (make a batch for the next few days)
Snack: Mushroom Madness (page 212)
Yoga: Heart-Pumping Sweaty Flow (page 119)
Dinner: Indian Curry Mix (page 233)
Dessert: Peanut Butter Cookie Bars
Evening Meditation: Calm Eyes (page 162)

DAY 14

Morning Meditation: one minute of Breath of Fire (page 159), followed by four minutes of Easy Breathing (page 155)

Breakfast: Granola (page 189) (make a big batch for the week) + The Swamp (page 181)

Yoga: Heart-Pumping Sweaty Flow (page 119)

Lunch: Cheesy Kale Rice (page 240)

Snack: Fresh Guacamole (page 197) with veggies + Turn Up the Beet (page 171)

Yoga: Body Awareness Flow (page 107)

Dinner: Tomato Cream Soup

Dessert: Banana Soft Serve (page 248)

Evening Meditation: five minutes of Bellows Breathing (page 160)

DAY 15

Morning Meditation: five minutes of Easy Breathing (page 155)

Breakfast: Maple French Toast (page 193)

Yoga: Body Awareness Flow (page 107)

Lunch: Tomato Cream Soup

Snack: Strawberry Shortcake Smoothie (page 185)

Yoga: Easygoing Winding Down the Evening Flow (page 138)

Dinner: Steamed Kale with a Kick (page 225) + Candied Sweet Potato Fries (page 224)

Dessert: Ice-Cream Sandwiches (page 249)
Evening Meditation: five minutes of Alternate Nostril Breathing (page 156)

DAY 16
Morning Meditation: five minutes of 4 Count Breathing (page 156)
Breakfast: Granola + Turn Up the Beet (page 171)
Yoga: Body Awareness Flow (page 107)
Lunch: Kale Krunch (page 213)
Snack: Savory & Spicy Mushroom Bites (page 196)
Yoga: Easygoing Winding Down the Evening Flow (page 138)
Dinner: Energy Bowl (page 239)
Dessert: Snickerdoodles (page 247) (make a batch for the next few days and to share with friends)
Evening Meditation: two minutes of Hug the Universe (page 158)

DAY 17
Morning Meditation: one minute of Breath of Fire (page 159)
Breakfast: Banango (page 177)
Yoga: Energizing Morning Flow (page 80)
Lunch: Freggies (page 211)
Snack: Aloha Dreams (page 173)
Yoga: Heart-Pumping Sweaty Flow (page 119)
Dinner: Fire Bowl (page 237)

Dessert: Snickerdoodles
Evening Meditation: five minutes of 4 Count Breathing (page 156)
DAY 18
Morning Meditation: five minutes of Alternate Nostril Breathing (page 156)
Breakfast: Granola + The Popeye (page 172)
Yoga: Heart-Pumping Sweaty Flow (page 119)
Lunch: Mexican Chilled Wrap (page 217)
Snack: Fresh Guacamole (page 197) with veggies
Yoga: Body Awareness Flow (page 107)
Dinner: Steamed Kale with a Kick (page 225) + Mashed Sweet Potatoes (page 223)
Dessert: Ice-Cream Sandwich (page 249)
Evening Meditation: five minutes of Bellows Breathing (page 160)
DAY 19
Morning Meditation: one minute of Breath of Fire (page 159)
Breakfast: Chocolate Almond Butter Protein Bomb (page 183)
Yoga: Craving Control Flow (page 98)
Lunch: Chopt & Spicy (page 209)
Snack: Granola
Yoga: Body Awareness Flow (page 107)
Dinner: All Veggies in My Burrito (page 218)

Dessert: Warm Chocolate Berry Bowl (page 251)
Evening Meditation: five minutes of 4 Count Breathing (page 156)

DAY 20
Morning Meditation: five minutes of Alternate Nostril Breathing (page 156)
Breakfast: Banango (page 177)
Yoga: Energizing Morning Flow (page 80)
Lunch: Roasted Acorn Squash Soup (page 207) (make a batch for the next few days)
Snack: Mushroom Madness (page 212)
Yoga: Body Awareness Flow (page 107)
Dinner: Portobello Burger Heaven (page 231) + Candied Sweet Potato Fries (page 224)
Dessert: Banana Soft Serve (page 248)
Evening Meditation: five minutes of Mantra Meditation (page 160)

DAY 21
Morning Meditation: five minutes of Easy Breathing (page 155)
Breakfast: The Swamp (page 181)
Yoga: Heart-Pumping Sweaty Flow (page 119)
Lunch: Kale Krunch (page 213)
Snack: Roasted Acorn Squash Soup
Yoga: Easygoing Winding Down the Evening Flow (page 138)

Dinner: Shells & Cheese (page 235) (make a big batch for the next few days)
Dessert: Ice-Cream Sandwich (page 249)
Evening Meditation: five minutes of Bellows Breathing (page 160)
DAY 22
Morning Meditation: five minutes of 4 Count Breathing (page 156)
Breakfast: Chocolate Almond Butter Protein Bomb (page 183)
Yoga: Heart-Pumping Sweaty Flow (page 119)
Lunch: Shells & Cheese
Snack: Spicy Avocado Toast (page 191)
Yoga: Easy Mind Calm Body Flow (page 114)
Dinner: Indian Curry Mix (page 233)
Dessert: Warm Chocolate Berry Bowl (page 251)
Evening Meditation: Calm Eyes (page 162)
DAY 23
Morning Meditation: one minute of Breath of Fire (page 159)
Breakfast: Granola (page 189) (make a big batch for the week) + Turn Up the Beet (page 171)
Yoga: Heart-Pumping Sweaty Flow (page 119)
Lunch: Mashed Sweet Potatoes (page 223) + Spinach and Quinoa Delight (page 228)
Snack: Savory & Spicy Mushroom Bites (page 196)

Yoga: Body Awareness Flow (page 107)
Dinner: Shells & Cheese
Dessert: Healthy Frosty (page 178)
Evening Meditation: five minutes of Mantra Meditation (page 160)
DAY 24
Morning Meditation: five minutes of 4 Count Breathing (page 156)
Breakfast: Spicy Avocado Toast (page 191)
Yoga: Body Awareness Flow (page 107)
Lunch: Shells & Cheese
Snack: Thin Mints Girl Scout Smoothie (page 179)
Yoga: Heart-Pumping Sweaty Flow (page 119)
Dinner: All Veggies in My Burrito (page 218)
Dessert: Strawberry Shortcake Smoothie (page 185)
Evening Meditation: five minutes of Mantra Meditation (page 160)
DAY 25
Morning Meditation: five minutes of Easy Breathing (page 155)
Breakfast: Granola + Green River (page 170)
Yoga: Easy Mind Calm Body Flow (page 114)
Lunch: Fresh Guacamole (page 197) with veggies + Kale Krunch (page 213)
Snack: Aloha Dreams (page 173)

Yoga: Easygoing Winding Down the Evening Flow (page 138)
Dinner: Energy Bowl (page 239)
Dessert: Warm Chocolate Berry Bowl (page 251)
Evening Meditation: five minutes of Alternate Nostril Breathing (page 156)
DAY 26
Morning Meditation: two minutes of Hug the Universe (page 158)
Breakfast: Spicy Avocado Toast (page 191) + The Popeye (page 172)
Yoga: Energizing Morning Flow (page 80)
Lunch: Roasted Acorn Squash Soup (page 207) (make a batch for the next few days)
Snack: Healthy Frosty (page 178)
Yoga: Craving Control Flow (page 98)
Dinner: Fire Bowl (page 237)
Dessert: Warm Chocolate Berry Bowl (page 251)
Evening Meditation: two minutes of Hug the Universe (page 158)
DAY 27
Morning Meditation: five minutes of Alternate Nostril Breathing (page 156)
Breakfast: Banango (page 177)
Yoga: Energizing Morning Flow (page 80)
Lunch: Roasted Acorn Squash Soup

Snack: Freggies (page 211)
Yoga: Body Awareness Flow (page 107)
Dinner: Cheesy Kale Rice (page 240)
Dessert: Almond Butter Fudge (page 243) (make a batch for the next few days)
Evening Meditation: five minutes of Easy Breathing (page 155)
DAY 28
Morning Meditation: five minutes of 4 Count Breathing (page 156)
Breakfast: Strawberry Shortcake Smoothie (page 185)
Yoga: Body Awareness Flow (page 107)
Lunch: Roasted Acorn Squash Soup
Snack: Granola (page 189)
Yoga: Easygoing Winding Down the Evening Flow (page 138)
Dinner: Indian Curry Mix (page 233)
Dessert: Almond Butter Fudge
Evening Meditation: five minutes of Bellows Breathing (page 160)
DAY 29
Morning Meditation: five minutes of Easy Breathing (page 155)
Breakfast: Hot Fruit Bowl (page 190)
Yoga: Body Awareness Flow (page 107)

Lunch: Spinach and Quinoa Delight (page 228)
Snack: Spicy Avocado Toast (page 191)
Yoga: Easy Mind Calm Body Flow (page 114)
Dinner: Spicy Sautéed Mushroom and Kale (page 227) + Mashed Sweet Potatoes (page 223)
Dessert: Almond Butter Fudge
Evening Meditation: five minutes of Mantra Meditation (page 160)
DAY 30
Morning Meditation: one minute of Breath of Fire (page 159)
Breakfast: Maple French Toast (page 193)
Yoga: Craving Control Flow (page 98)
Lunch: Chopt & Spicy (page 209)
Snack: Spinach Cashew Mix (page 195)
Yoga: Body Awareness Flow (page 107)
Dinner: Energy Bowl (page 239)
Dessert: Almond Butter Fudge
Evening Meditation: Calm Eyes (page 162)

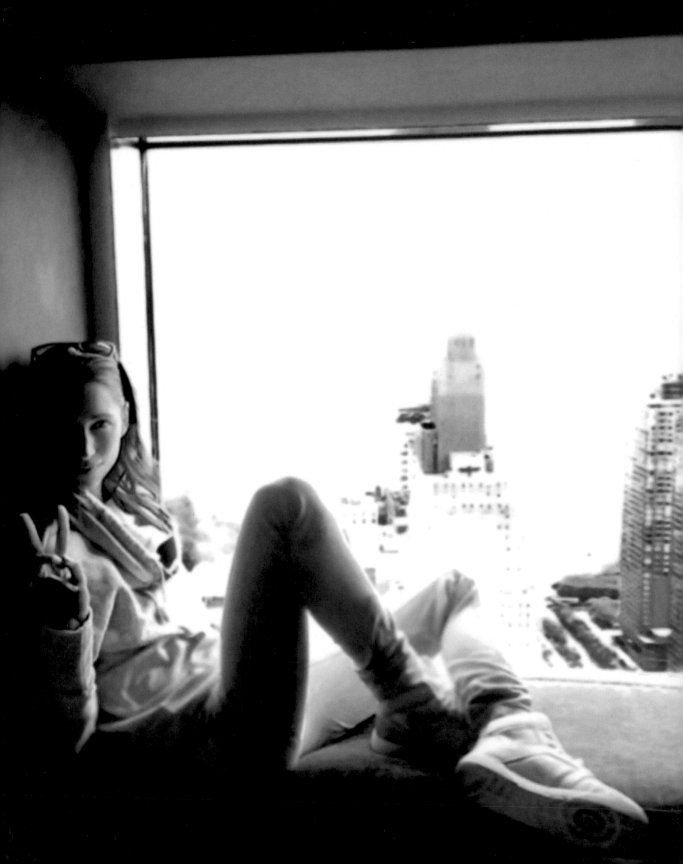

final wishes for you

Congratulations! You've made it. And as I leave you on your way to creating an amazing life, I will just remind you of the one thing you always need to remember: you are already perfect. All the work you do is to keep you connected to believing that. Don't believe anyone who tells you differently. Don't believe your mind when it tries to convince you otherwise. I used to go through life thinking and comparing myself with others. I used to measure myself, weigh myself, criticize myself, and restrict myself. I felt tense, judged, angry, and isolated.

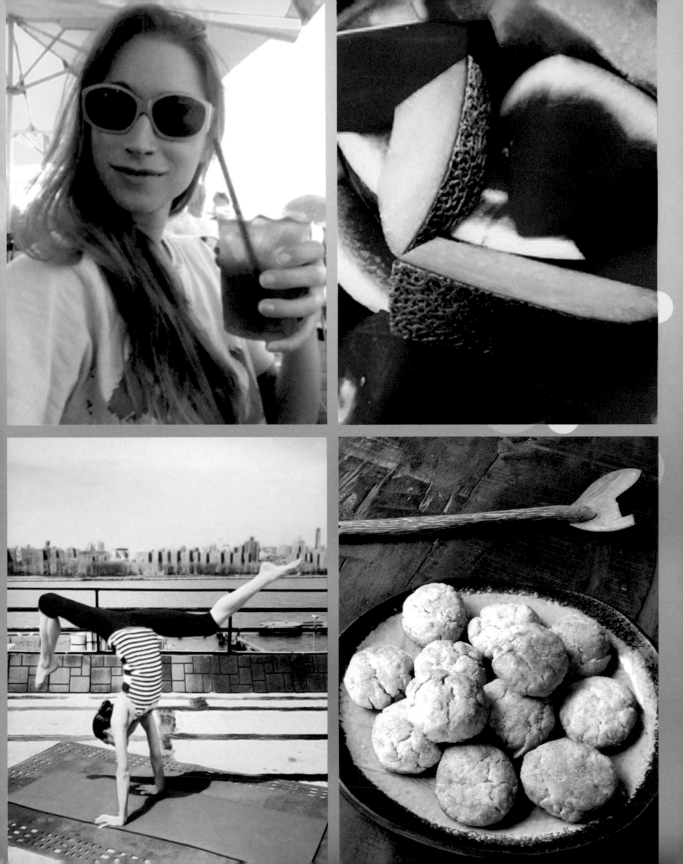

I embodied tension, and that's what came back at me. I was frustrated that I wasn't getting the results I wanted in my life.

After too long practicing what didn't work, I decided to practice something else. Not only did I give myself permission to feel, I also gave myself permission to believe what I feel and respond to it. I no longer measure, weigh, or criticize. I feel at ease, open, connected, and happy. My life is expansive, and it flows with ease. I am able to handle stress without getting boxed in. I am able to navigate and experience the spontaneous joy that life offers. I am able to fully express myself. In moments when I feel disconnected, I know how to get reconnected, and I decide to practice. I continue to practice.

I know the information in this book works, and I know it will work for you. You simply need to begin now. Don't procrastinate. Start right now.

I deeply desire that you give yourself permission to feel and to create habits that make you feel fantastic. You can do it, and I'm rooting for you big-time.

Remember, there is nothing for you to fix; you're just reconnecting to who you truly are. By doing this, you can be ridiculously happy. And when you're happy, you can't help but make other people happy. I want you to become this model of health and happiness so you can guide everyone you meet into radiant, ridiculous happiness, too.

Everything you need to guide you to live a fantastic, radiant life is within you. The routines, the yoga, the meditation, the cooking—these are all just things that will help keep you connected. The goal is to take care of yourself so you can live a meaningful, purposeful, and enjoyable life. Allow yourself to go along for the ride and have fun.

ENJOY!

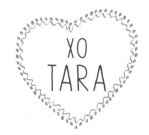

XO
TARA

acknowledgments

Thank you to the heads of nourishment in my family.

Mom, Dad, Grandma Gray, Grandma Richardson, Aunt Mary, Rindy Sharon, and Tony, you kept me alive and well and taught me about food, family, and loving time together around the kitchen.

Thank you to everyone at Strala NYC and global who keeps the community nourished and healthy and expanding. Gratitude to Anna Gannon, Jennifer Grossi, Sophie Blanco, Sandrine Bridoux, Cindy Xu, Suzy Sorenson, Vera Boykevich, Humberto Cruz, Jes Allen, Kati Rediger, Shawn Li, and the team for your patience, support, occasional taste testing, and honest feedback.

Thank you to Will Hobbs for the support all these years. Patty Gift, Richelle Zizian, Erin Dupree, thank you for welcoming me into the Hay House family, your guidance, and pushing.

Thank you to Laura Gray for all your time, patience, thoughtful contributions, and loads of laughs.

Thank you to Andrew Scrivani for your awesome photography and creativity. I'm so happy you actually ate and enjoyed all the healthy meals I made.

Thank you to Ryan Kibler for the fresh cover photo and Anja Grasseger for always being there when I need a refresher.

Thank you to Liang Shi for awesome designs and inspiration.

Thank you to Charles McStravick for the superinspired fun design and layout, jumping on board with my wacky ideas, and improving them a ton.

Thank you to Dr. Mark Hyman for your generous foreword and support. You rock, my friend.

Thank you to Kris Carr, Tia Mowry, Jessica Ortner, Gabby Bernstein, Latham Thomas, and the Crazy Sexy family of supporters.

Thank you to my partners at Reebok and W for all the support.

And finally, thank you to the people who practice Strala around the world, readers of my blog and books, viewers of my videos, and everyone who has shared your story with me, whether in person at a workshop, randomly on the street, or in a sweet note. This process is about connecting, sharing, and expanding. We are co-creating and healing ourselves and one another together. Thank you.

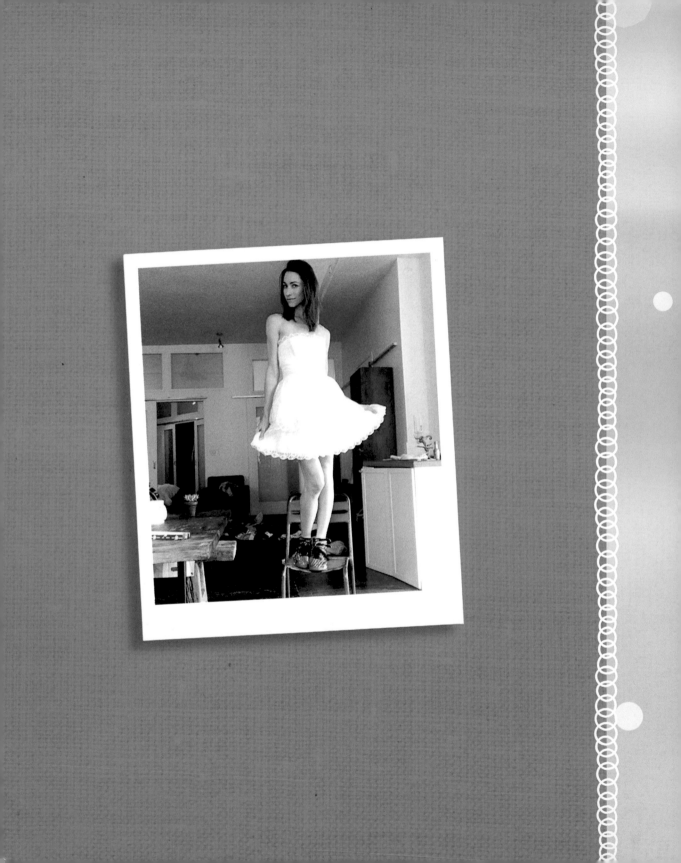

about the author

Named "Yoga Rebel" by The New York Times, Tara Stiles is the founder and owner of Strala, the movement system that ignites freedom and is widely known for its unpretentious, inclusive, and straightforward approach to yoga and meditation. Tara has also been profiled by *The New York Times, The Times of India, The Times* (UK), and *Dagens Nyheter,* and featured in many major national and international magazines.

Tara is the designer and face of Reebok's yoga lifestyle line and author of two best-selling books: *Slim Calm Sexy Yoga* and *Yoga Cures.* She has created several DVD collaborations with Jane Fonda, Deepak Chopra, Tia Mowry, Brooklyn Decker, and *ELLE* magazine. In addition, the Alliance for a Healthier Generation, Bill Clinton's initiative to combat childhood obesity, tapped Tara to help promote activity to 21,000-plus participating schools.

Jane Fonda named Tara "the new face of fitness," and *Vanity Fair* declared her the "Coolest Yoga Instructor Ever."

Visit www.tarastiles.com.

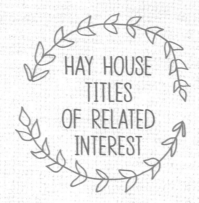

HAY HOUSE TITLES OF RELATED INTEREST

YOU CAN HEAL YOUR LIFE, the movie, starring Louise Hay & Friends
(available as a 1-DVD program and an expanded 2-DVD set)
Watch the trailer at: www.LouiseHayMovie.com

THE SHIFT, the movie, starring Dr. Wayne W. Dyer
(available as a 1-DVD program and an expanded 2-DVD set)
Watch the trailer at: www.DyerMovie.com

CRAZY SEXY KITCHEN:
150 Plant-Empowered Recipes to Ignite a Mouthwatering Revolution,
by Kris Carr with Chef Chad Sarno

LOVING YOURSELF TO GREAT HEALTH:
Thoughts & Food—The Ultimate Diet,
by Louise Hay, Ahlea Khadro, and Heather Dane

MIRACLES NOW:
108 Life-Changing Tools for Less Stress, More Flow, and Finding Your True Purpose,
by Gabrielle Bernstein

SLIMMING MEALS THAT HEAL:
Lose Weight Without Dieting, Using Anti-inflammatory Superfoods,
by Julie Daniluk, R.H.N.

All of the above are available at your local bookstore,
or may be ordered by contacting Hay House (see next page).

WE HOPE YOU ENJOYED THIS HAY HOUSE BOOK. IF YOU'D LIKE TO RECEIVE
OUR ONLINE CATALOG FEATURING ADDITIONAL INFORMATION ON HAY HOUSE BOOKS AND PRODUCTS,
OR IF YOU'D LIKE TO FIND OUT MORE ABOUT THE HAY FOUNDATION, PLEASE CONTACT:

Hay House, Inc., P.O. Box 5100, Carlsbad, CA 92018-5100
(760) 431-7695 or (800) 654-5126
(760) 431-6948 (fax) or (800) 650-5115 (fax)
www.hayhouse.com® · www.hayfoundation.org

Published and distributed in Australia by:
Hay House Australia Pty. Ltd., 18/36 Ralph St., Alexandria NSW 2015
Phone: 612-9669-4299 · Fax: 612-9669-4144 · www.hayhouse.com.au

Published and distributed in the United Kingdom by:
Hay House UK, Ltd., Astley House, 33 Notting Hill Gate, London W11 3JQ
Phone: 44-20-3675-2450 · Fax: 44-20-3675-2451 · www.hayhouse.co.uk

Published and distributed in the Republic of South Africa by:
Hay House SA (Pty.), Ltd., P.O. Box 990, Witkoppen 2068
Phone/Fax: 27-11-467-8904 · www.hayhouse.co.za

Published in India by:
Hay House Publishers India, Muskaan Complex, Plot No. 3, B-2, Vasant Kunj, New Delhi 110 070
Phone: 91-11-4176-1620 · Fax: 91-11-4176-1630 · www.hayhouse.co.in

Distributed in Canada by:
Raincoast Books, 2440 Viking Way, Richmond, B.C. V6V 1N2
Phone: 1-800-663-5714 · Fax: 1-800-565-3770 · www.raincoast.com

Visit www.HealYourLife.com® to regroup, recharge, and reconnect with your own magnificence.
Featuring blogs, mind-body-spirit news, and life-changing wisdom from Louise Hay and friends.

Visit www.HealYourLife.com today!

FREE E-NEWSLETTERS FROM HAY HOUSE, THE ULTIMATE RESOURCE FOR INSPIRATION

Be the first to know about Hay House's dollar deals, free downloads, special offers, affirmation cards, giveaways, contests, and more!

 Get exclusive excerpts from our latest releases and videos from *Hay House Present Moments*.

 Enjoy uplifting personal stories, how-to articles, and healing advice, along with videos and empowering quotes, within *Heal Your Life*.

 Have an inspirational story to tell and a passion for writing? Sharpen your writing skills with insider tips from *Your Writing Life*.

Sign Up Now!

Get inspired, educate yourself, get a complimentary gift, and share the wisdom!

http://www.hayhouse.com/newsletters.php

Visit www.hayhouse.com to sign up today!

HAY HOUSE

HAYHOUSE RADIO
radio for your soul™

HealYourLife.com

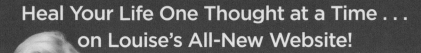

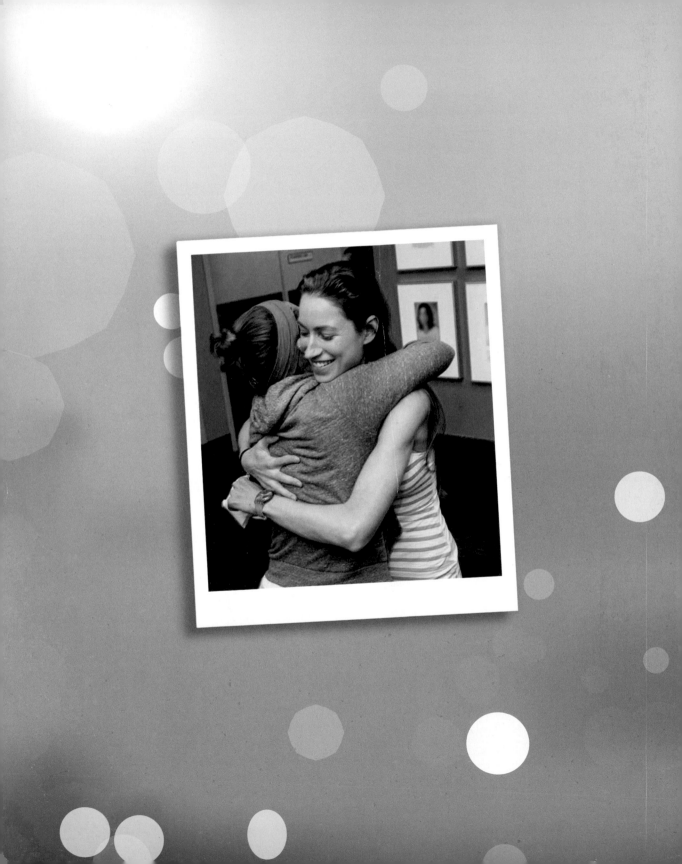